618.1
Lar

W9-DHS-303

The Estrogen Decision

A Self-Help Program

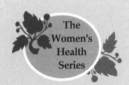

The Women's Health Series

SUSAN M. LARK, M.D.

Westchester Publishing Company
Los Altos, California

Middlebury Community
Library

Cover & Text Design: Brad Greene
Photographs: Ronald May
Illustrations: Shelly Reeves Smith
Printing & Binding: Arcata Graphics/Kingsport

Copyright © 1994 by Susan M. Lark, M.D.

Manufactured in the United States of America.
All rights reserved. No portion of this book may be
reproduced in any form, except for brief review,
without written permission of the publisher.
International Standard Book Number: 0-917010-56-6
Library of Congress Catalog Card Number: 93-60454

𝒲estchester Publishing Company
342 State Street, Suite 6
Los Altos, CA 94022
415-941-5784

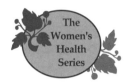

The Women's Health Series

Anemia and Heavy Menstrual Flow
Menstrual Cramps
Chronic Fatigue and Tiredness
Fibroid Tumors and Endometriosis
Anxiety and Stress
The Estrogen Decision

Middlebury Community
Library

Contents

To my wonderful husband Jim and
my darling daughter Rebecca
To the health and well-being of all women

NOTE: The information in this book is meant to complement the advice and guidance of your physician, not replace it. It is very important that women experiencing menopausal symptoms have these problems evaluated by a physician. If you are under the care of a physician, you should discuss any major changes in your regimen with him or her. Because this is a book and not a medical consultation, keep in mind that the information presented here may not apply in your particular case. In view of individual medical requirements, new research, and government regulations, it is the responsibility of the reader to validate health practices and treatment with a physician or health service.

Introduction

$\mathcal{M}$illions of women today face a major decision whether or not to use estrogen during and after menopause. They include not only women who have ceased menstruating entirely, but also women in their forties and early fifties whose age and menstrual cycle changes indicate the approach of menopause. Menopause, by definition, means the last menstrual period, but many people use the term more loosely to include the years leading up to and following the last period. The number of women facing this important decision is growing dramatically as the large population increase of women born after World War II reaches midlife. In fact, the number of women between the ages of 45 to 54 is expected to grow 73 percent between 1990 and 2010, according to a recent article published in *American Demographics* (35 million women in the United States are currently menopausal). For women in their menopausal and postmenopausal years, the maintenance of good health and well-being, as well as prevention of diseases of aging such as heart disease and cancer, become major issues. The role of estrogen in attaining these goals is a central issue for most midlife women.

How Women Differ in Their Need for Estrogen

I have been dealing with the estrogen issue in my medical practice for nearly twenty years. As a physician specializing in women's health care and preventive medicine, I have heard numerous questions from concerned women about the efficacy and safety of estrogen.

This decision has no "one right answer." Each menopausal woman is different. Some women with severe symptoms such as hot flashes, night sweats, vaginal dryness or mood swings can certainly benefit from the use of estrogen. Other women choose to use estrogen to prevent longer-term health problems, such as osteoporosis and heart disease, for which they are at risk. These women feel strongly about the benefits of using estrogen and tolerate the hormonal therapy well.

Unfortunately, many women deviate from this "ideal" pattern of good acceptance and tolerance of estrogen therapy. Some women, together with their physician or on their own, make the choice not to take estrogen. This decision may be due to the fact that estrogen replacement therapy could intensify serious pre-existing health problems such as uterine cancer, heavy bleeding from uterine fibroid tumors, severe migraine headaches, or blood clotting problems. Other women, free of illness, fear that the long-term use of estrogen may accelerate onset of a disease for which they are at risk, based on a strong family history. This concern occurs most often among women whose mothers or sisters have had breast cancer. Other women would like to use estrogen but experience unacceptable side effects such as depression, breast tenderness, or fluid retention that occur no matter how the estrogen is given or at what dosage. Approximately 20 percent of menopausal women in developed countries like the United States have no menopause symptoms or their symptoms are so mild that they manage well without estrogen therapy. Some women refuse to use estrogen on a philosophical basis, even if they could benefit from it, preferring instead to pursue nondrug treatment options such as nutritional therapies and acupuncture. As you may conclude, the decision of whether or not to take estrogen is a very complicated one and should not be made without knowing all the facts.

Women's Needs are Often Not Met

Unfortunately, health care researchers and providers have done very little to accommodate the needs of these diverse groups of women. Most often, a woman with menopausal symptoms goes to her physician and hears that she may either choose hormonal replacement therapy or not. Few learn about alternative therapies and even fewer hear how to use lifestyle modification to reduce menopausal symptoms and risk factors for disease. As a result, many women do not get the treatment best suited to their needs. A 1994 Gallup Poll indicated that 40 percent (with a margin of error of 2 to 4 percentage points) of menopausal women in the United States use estrogen replacement therapy. With 80 to 85 percent of all menopausal women symptomatic to some degree, many women who could benefit from estrogen treatment are either not receiving it or are seeking alternatives to traditional medical therapy. Many women are uninformed concerning the treatment options available to them or they are uncertain about the right path to choose.

The Purpose of This Book

I have written this book to help demystify the various menopause treatments, both estrogen replacement therapy (ERT) and alternative therapies. I wish to share with you and other women the many treatment options that can produce effective menopause relief. A woman need not choose one option to the exclusion of all others. By looking at each woman's current state of health, lifestyle habits, family health background, and risk factors for various diseases, a health care provider can almost always develop an effective menopause-relief program. In my practice, many patients choose to use estrogen in its many different forms and dose regimens; however, they usually combine it with healthful dietary changes and improved exercise habits, as well as learning how to handle day-to-day stress better. Often they are far healthier using both ERT and lifestyle modification than they could ever be following only one treatment option. Patients who cannot or do not choose to use estrogen also do well with an alternative therapy program. Later in the book, I shall discuss alternative programs to protect the heart, bones and emotional well-being of a woman when she does not take ERT.

To help you develop the best treatment program for yourself, included in this book is much of the information I have shared over the years with women who have seen me as patients or attended my classes. You will find the most useful and recent research on the pros and cons of estrogen therapy. I also discuss the health benefits of lifestyle modification for menopause symptom-relief. (Unlike the research on estrogen, very little of the research on topics such as diet, nutritional supplements and exercise ever reach the consumer, the women who could really benefit from this knowledge.) Also included are helpful tips and practical guidelines for easily and simply instituting healthful lifestyle changes. After reading this book, be sure to share with your health care practitioner any questions you have about ERT or other therapies. If you do not feel that your doctor is receptive to your concerns and questions, you may have to find another practitioner in your community with whom you feel more comfortable to meet your needs. Ideally, doctor and patient should work together as a team on the patient's behalf, implementing the best solutions to the patient's health care problems. To achieve this goal, you may have to assume an active role and take responsibility for letting your physician know that you wish to participate in the process of making decisions about your health and well-being. You may also need to convey that it is important to you to have meaningful dialogue about important issues.

How to Use This Book

This book is divided into two parts to make it easy and effective to use. Part I contains a chapter on the basic facts about female hormones: how we produce and metabolize estrogen in our body and how this process changes as we go through menopause. The role estrogen (and the other female hormone, progesterone) plays in helping to maintain the body's state of health is the first focus. In the remainder of Part I, estrogen replacement therapy (ERT) is covered in detail, including information on the different types and dosages of ERT as well as other hormones used for menopause treatment. Information is included on who should use ERT, as well as the short- and long-term benefits and the controversies surrounding its use.

In Part II, alternative treatments for specific menopausal symptoms are covered. Chapters on diet, vitamins, minerals, essential fatty acids and herbs are included as well as sections on acupressure, yoga, physical exercise and stress reduction techniques.

Discuss the ERT treatment option with your physician to see if it makes sense for you. If you decide not to use estrogen after considering the risks, try the alternative therapies for symptom relief described in the book. Many of my patients have combined ERT and alternative treatments with very positive results. Above all, remember that information contained in this book is presented to help you make educated choices about your health care needs. When you are knowledgeable and informed, you are far more likely to make choices that will bring you symptom relief and better health. Your midlife years and beyond can be exciting and fulfilling when you participate actively in your health care decisions.

Hormone Replacement Therapy: Is it for You ?

❖   ❖   ❖

What is Estrogen?

$\mathcal{A}$ woman's body produces three hormones that support the normal functioning of the reproductive tract and menstrual cycle. These powerful hormones help regulate not only body chemistry but physical characteristics such as skin texture, muscle tone and body shape. The two female hormones that we make in substantial amounts during our active childbearing years are estrogen and progesterone. We also make very small amounts of male hormones, androgens, that affect our female functions. An example of such a hormone is testosterone. This chapter will discuss these hormones and their role in female development.

What Are Hormones?

Hormones are chemicals secreted by glands in the body. Once a hormone is released into the bloodstream, it may circulate to a target gland. The hormone acts as a messenger, instructing the target gland to make its own hormone. In some instances, a hormone triggers chemical reactions in different parts of the body. The body makes dozens of hormones, most of which are outside the scope of this book, because they regulate functions unrelated to the reproductive system. For example, some hormones regulate how efficiently we can fight off viral and bacterial infections, while others regulate digestive processes. Still other hormones help our bodies manage stressful situations effectively by regulating muscle tension and blood flow to vital organs.

Certain glands such as the ovaries, adrenals, pituitary and hypothalamus assume a major role in producing and regulating levels of the three hormones estrogen, progesterone and androgens. These hormones regulate the menstrual cycle and later in life, determine how easily we transition through menopause. Other glands, such as the thyroid, also play a supporting role. Let us look at how they produce our female hormones, first during our active reproductive years and then how this process changes as we approach menopause.

Hormone Production During the Menstrual Cycle

We begin by discussing the normal menstrual cycle and how it functions. This information will help you understand the normal ebb and flow of our female hormones throughout the month.

First, let's understand why menstruation occurs. Menstruation refers to the shedding of the uterine lining, or endometrium. Each month the uterus prepares a thick, blood-rich cushion to nourish and house a fertilized egg. If conception occurs, the embryo implants itself in the uterine lining after six or seven days. If pregnancy does not occur, the egg does not implant in the uterus and the extra buildup of uterine lining is not needed. The uterus cleanses itself by releasing the extra blood and tissue so the buildup can recur the following month.

The mechanism that regulates the buildup and shedding of the uterine lining is controlled by fluctuations in hormonal levels. These fluctuations are based on a feedback system. When the ovaries secrete high levels of estrogen and progesterone, this "turns off" production of hypothalamic and pituitary hormones that normally stimulate ovarian function. Conversely, when ovarian production of estrogen and progesterone are low, the hypothalamic and pituitary hormone production rises in an attempt to stimulate the ovaries to work harder.

How does the feedback system operate in the menstrual cycle? The initial trigger for the menstrual cycle comes from hormones produced in the hypothalamus, a walnut-sized collection of highly specialized brain cells located above the pituitary. The hypothalamus regulates many basic bodily functions in addition to the production of female sex hormones, including temperature control, sleep patterns, thirst and hunger. The hypothalamus is very sensitive to stress such as emotional problems and infections. Severe stress can affect the ability of the hypothalamus to pass signals to the pituitary and on to the other endocrine glands. This can cause an imbalance in the menstrual cycle.

The pituitary, located at the base of the brain, stimulates all the glands of the body and provides the next mechanism that regulates the menstrual cycle. To communicate with the pituitary, the hypothalamus releases messengers into the bloodstream called FSH-RF (follicle-stimulating hormone-releasing factor) and LH-RF (luteinizing hormone-releasing factor). When these messages from the hypothalamus are received, the pituitary begins to produce its own hormones which trigger the menstrual cycle and ovulation by secreting FSH (follicle-stimulating hormone) and LH (luteinizing hormone). The pituitary also triggers adrenal function through the production of ACTH (adrenocorticotrophic hormone) and thyroid function through TSH (thyroid-stimulating hormone).

Once FSH and LH are released into the bloodstream, their destinations are the ovaries, the female reproductive organ. The ovaries are two small, almond-shaped glands located in a woman's pelvis. The ovaries hold all the eggs a woman will ever have, in an inactive form called follicles. At birth, each female may have as many as 1 million follicles. By puberty, the number of eggs has been reduced to 300,000 to 400,000. The eggs decrease in number throughout a woman's life, until menopause, at which time the follicles have atrophied and lost their ability to produce estrogen. Without sufficient estrogen, menstruation ceases.

Each month, FSH and LH from the pituitary cause the follicles to ripen and the release of an egg for possible fertilization. (Usually only one ovary is stimulated in a cycle.) In doing so, the follicles begin to produce the hormones estrogen and progesterone. Estrogen reaches its peak during the first half of the cycle, while progesterone output occurs after midcycle when ovulation has occurred.

Following menstruation, during the first half of the menstrual cycle, the endometrium or uterine lining gradually rebuilds itself. Estrogen causes the glands of the endometrium to begin to grow long; the lining thickens through an increase in the number of blood vessels, as well as the production of a mesh of fibers that interconnect throughout the lining. By midcycle, the lining of the uterus has increased three times in thickness and has a greatly increased blood supply.

After midcycle, usually around day 14 in a 28-day cycle, ovulation occurs. Ovulation refers to the production of a mature egg cell which is capable of being fertilized. Normally, the mature egg finds its way to a fallopian tube for the journey to the uterus. The follicle that produced the egg for that month (or Graafian follicle) is further stimulated after midcycle by LH and changes into the yellow body, or corpus luteum. The corpus luteum secretes progesterone—the second ovarian hormone of the menstrual cycle. Progesterone helps prepare the uterine lining for a possible pregnancy. With stimulation by progesterone, the uterine lining secretes glycogen (a storage form of sugar), mucous, and other substances needed to sustain a fertilized egg. Progesterone also causes a coiling of the blood vessels and the uterine lining becomes swollen and tortuous.

If the egg is fertilized, it will implant on the uterine wall and the corpus luteum will continue to secrete progesterone. If no fertilization occurs, the corpus luteum begins to deteriorate and the progesterone and estrogen levels decrease. The lining of the uterus starts to break down and menstruation begins. With the onset of menstruation, the monthly ebb and flow of hormones begins again.

Hormone Balance in the Body

When the levels of estrogen and progesterone are optimally balanced throughout the month, female menstrual and reproductive health is the result. However, optimal function not only depends on how much of each hormone is produced, but also on how efficiently the body metabolizes and disposes of the hormones. Once they have done their job, they no longer need to remain in the body. Normally, the hormones are metabolized and broken down by the liver. This occurs as they pass through the liver while circulating in the bloodstream. For example, when liver function is healthy and efficient it will transform the main type of estrogen secreted by the ovary, called estradiol, into other forms of estrogen. Estradiol is a chemically active and efficient form of estrogen. It binds to many tissues such as the uterus, breasts and ovaries, as well as the brain, heart and other organ systems in the body through specific estrogen receptors that allow it to enter into the cells. As a potent form of estrogen, estradiol stimulates many chemical reactions in the target tissues.

However, as with everything in life, proper balance is important. When estradiol is present in too high an amount or for too prolonged a period of time, it can cause adverse reactions in the body. Research studies suggest that, when unopposed, it may be carcinogenic to estrogen-sensitive tissues such as the breast and uterus. The liver prevents excessive build-up of estradiol in the blood circulation by inactivating it. The liver converts estradiol to a less active, intermediary form called estrone and finally to estriol, a very weak form of estrogen. Like estradiol, these weaker forms of estrogen can also bind to estrogen receptors in the cells. However, their physiological effect on the body is less pronounced. Although estrone is also a carcinogenic form of estrogen, medical research studies suggest that estriol may actually decrease our susceptibility toward developing female-related cancers such as breast cancer. Estradiol is 12 times more potent than estrone and 80 times more potent than estriol. Thus, the total estrogenic effect of estradiol is many times greater than the other two forms combined; therefore, smaller doses are needed.

When the liver is healthy, the conversion process occurs quite efficiently. However, poor nutritional habits can compromise healthy liver function. The intake of too much alcohol, fat or sugar can impair the liver's ability to handle the overload of food as well as the breakdown of the female hormones. In addition, research studies have shown that a lack of sufficient B vitamins adversely affects estrogen metabolism.

Estrogen passes from the liver via the bile into the intestinal tract. Again, diet affects how estrogen is handled in the intestinal tract. When a woman eats a high-fat, low-fiber diet, the dietary fat stimulates the growth of certain types of bacteria in the intestinal tract. These bacteria chemically change the breakdown products of estrogen into forms that can be reabsorbed back into the body. As with poor liver function, this process elevates the levels of estrone and estradiol in the bloodstream. In contrast, a low-fat, high-fiber diet promotes excretion of estrogen by the body. High dietary fiber binds with estrogen in the intestinal tract and helps remove it from the body in bowel movements. Estrogen is also excreted from the body through the urinary tract.

How Estrogen Affects the Body

As mentioned earlier, estrogen enters the cells of many different tissues and stimulates chemical reactions and physiological changes. Let us look at how estrogen affects our sexual organs and the physical characteristics that we tend to think of as specifically female. First of all, estrogen causes the growth of our sexual organs. During childhood, we produce estrogen in only small amounts. During puberty, estrogen productions increases twenty-fold or more. With the increased estrogenic stimulation, female sexual organs begin to change into those of adult women. Our uterus, vagina and fallopian tubes increase in size; our external genitals enlarge. Fat disposition occurs in the outer lips of the vulva (the labia majora). The smaller, inner lips (the labia minora) also enlarge. Our vaginal and urinary tract linings thicken and become much more resistant to trauma and infection. This is important in adulthood when women become sexually active. With estrogen stimulation, the lining of the uterus thickens and the endometrial glands develop—necessary to nourish a fertilized egg during the early stages of pregnancy.

In addition to causing maturation of the female sexual organs, estrogen causes an increase in overall body fat. This is particularly pronounced in the buttocks, hips and breasts, contributing to the softly rounded female contours that we associate with sexual maturation. Estrogen is responsible for the disposition of fat under the skin, giving rise to the soft and fine-textured skin that many women enjoy during their younger years. Estrogen also causes fluid and salt retention in the tissues, which additionally helps to plump up and fill out our skin.

Estrogen has an important effect on promoting bone health. It helps retain calcium in the bones thereby protecting against bone loss. By reducing the levels of low-density lipoprotein (LDL) in the body and elevating the levels of the protective blood fats, estrogen protects women from developing heart attacks and strokes. These "good" fats are called the high-density lipoproteins (HDL). Also, estrogen has a direct positive effect on the endothelial lining of the blood vessels, as well as affecting dozens of other physiological functions as varied as blood sugar level, emotional balance and memory.

How Progesterone Affects the Body

As mentioned earlier, progesterone is primarily produced by the corpus luteum (yellow body) of the ovary. It is also secreted in high doses by the placenta if a pregnancy occurs. Though estrogen primarily causes tissues to grow and thicken, progesterone has a maturing and growth-limiting effect on the tissues of the body. For example, progesterone prevents the uterine lining from thickening to the point where menstrual bleeding becomes too profuse and long lasting. Progesterone also stimulates secretory activity in the body. For example, under the stimulation of progesterone during the second half of the menstrual cycle, the uterine lining secretes nutrients needed by the developing embryo if pregnancy occurs. Progesterone also triggers the production of secretions in the fallopian tube. These secretions are important for the nutrition of the fertilized egg as it moves through the fallopian tube prior to implantation in the uterus. In breast tissue, progesterone causes certain cells to become secretory in their function which is necessary if the breasts are eventually to produce milk for nursing an infant.

The production of progesterone at midcycle causes an increase in body temperature by about one-half to one degree Fahrenheit. Many women monitor this temperature change to assess their fertility during the time of expected ovulation. Like estrogen, progesterone has an effect on many physical and chemical functions in the body. These effects often oppose and complement those of estrogen. For example, progesterone acts as a sedative on the nervous system. When progesterone levels are too high, it can cause depression and fatigue. In contrast, estrogen has a stimulatory effect on the nervous system. High levels of estrogen can trigger anxiety, irritability and mood swings. Progesterone tends to elevate the blood sugar level, while estrogen lowers it. Thus, the healthy balance between the two female hormones is very important.

How Androgens Affect the Body

As mentioned earlier, women secrete small amounts of androgens or male hormones. Both the ovaries and adrenal glands secrete small amounts of testosterone. Both of these glands manufacture testosterone from a precursor hormone called androstenedione. Like estrogen and progesterone, the level of androstenedione varies throughout the menstrual cycle.

The level rises at midcycle, when androstenedione is secreted from the ovarian follicle, and during the second half of the menstrual cycle when it is produced by the corpus luteum (which also secretes progesterone).

The secretion of small amounts of androgens are very important for female health. They help in maintaining our sex drive. Women who are placed on testosterone cream for various health problems or the oral estrogen/testosterone combination for HRT may note a significant increase in their sexual drive. Androgens also help maintain muscle strength as well as vaginal lubrication and elasticity. In fact, testosterone cream is sometimes applied directly to the vaginal tissues as a treatment for vaginal atrophy. It must be used carefully, however, because side effects of excessive androgen use can include masculinization such as deepening of the voice or growth of excessive facial hair.

Hormone Production During Menopause

As women reach their early forties, the reproductive tract begins to show signs of aging. By this time, most women have ovulated regularly for almost 30 years. With each ovulation, one follicle matures for a possible pregnancy. However, an additional 1000 follicles or more degenerate with each menstrual cycle and lose their ability to be fertilized. At this rate, most women have exhausted their supply of follicles by their late forties or early fifties.

As the number of follicles diminishes, the remaining follicles produce less estrogen. During the cycles when the follicles don't mature to ovulation, progesterone production is insufficient or absent. In fact, during the transition to menopause, ovulation occurs with decreasing frequency. Because of this drop in hormonal output by the ovaries, the pituitary hormone FSH rises in an attempt to drive the ovary to secrete more estrogen. Sometimes the high levels of FSH can overstimulate the remaining follicles to produce an abundance of estrogen. In such cycles, a woman may produce very high levels of estrogen yet not produce progesterone because the follicles never mature sufficiently. The tendency for estrogen to fluctuate between low and high levels of production can continue throughout the menopause transition and may last from one to seven years.

During this time, women are very vulnerable to developing a variety of health problems. The imbalance in the estrogen and progesterone levels can trigger the growth of uterine fibroids, PMS symptoms and changes in the amount and frequency of the menstrual cycle. Women whose estrogen level drops tend to have longer intervals between periods, with lighter bleeding, before stopping entirely. Women who have temporary surges in estrogen levels prior to menopause without the secretion of progesterone may have increasingly heavy and more frequent menstrual bleeding. The menstrual cycle often becomes irregular. This can be a very difficult time for some women and they are faced with the need for close monitoring by their physician when symptoms are severe. These symptoms present problems such as bleeding or fibroid growth which may lead to more hysterectomies in this age group.

Finally, as the follicles become exhausted, the estrogen drops to a level at which there is not enough of this hormone to build up the lining of the uterus sufficiently to induce menstruation. A woman is officially considered to be menopausal when she has had no menstrual period for at least six months. For most women, this occurs between the ages of 46 to 53. Some women, however, may experience menopause as early as their thirties or as late as age 59; the average age is 52.

As estrogen levels diminish, the level of FSH begins to rise, finally attaining levels considered to be diagnostic for menopause. FSH continues to remain high during the postmenopausal years. In fact, physicians often monitor FSH levels to determine the onset of menopause.

During the postmenopausal years, the body does continue to produce small amounts of estrogen. Even though the follicles are exhausted, another part of the ovary called the stroma can still make small amounts of estrogen. The stroma is the supportive tissue of the ovary that helps provide structure to the gland. In addition, the body can also make estrogen by converting the male precursor hormone, androstenedione, to estrogen. Though androstenedione is made by the adrenal glands, its conversion to estrogen occurs in the body's fat cells. Obese women make more estrogen after menopause because they have more fat cells. In fact, some women may make enough estrogen to delay aging of the skin, vagina, bladder, breasts, and other tissue for a decade or so. Thinner women tend to show loss of estrogen support earlier, as do women with less active adrenal or ovarian stromal output of hormones. By the time women reach their seventies and eighties, however, even these small extra sources of estrogen begin to diminish. As the hormonal support falls to lower and lower levels, the female body gradually ages during the years following menopause.

In the early postmenopausal years, common symptoms of diminished hormonal output include hot flashes, night sweats, vaginal and bladder atrophy, mood swings and fatigue. The lack of hormonal support can increase the risk of osteoporosis, heart attacks, adverse lipid and vessel wall changes, and stroke. These symptoms and health issues will be discussed in depth in the following chapters in terms of the treatment and prevention benefits estrogen replacement therapy (ERT) can provide.

2

Facts About Hormonal Replacement Therapy

$\mathcal{W}$hen you enter the early stages of menopause, the question of hormone replacement therapy (HRT) arises. The two female hormones, estrogen and progesterone (often in its synthetic version, the progestins), are certainly the most widely prescribed therapies utilized by physicians for the relief of menopausal symptoms and the prevention of certain hormone-related conditions of aging. Medical research during the past 50 years has created many different types and dosage regimens of hormones. Such therapies vary in terms of absorption, frequency of usage and dosage.

Many women are confused or uninformed about their choices of hormonal therapy. They don't know what to ask at medical visits to determine which hormonal regimens, if any, would suit them best. As a result, the best treatment combination for each individual woman may not be possible. Each woman should explore options and fine tune an individual approach until the best regimen is determined. This book will give you basic information about hormonal replacement therapy that can help you, with your physician, to make an intelligent and informed decision about using HRT. First, the history of hormonal replacement therapy in this country will be discussed; then, the steps to follow before beginning HRT. Detailed information is provided about the different types of estrogen, progesterone and even androgen therapy, as well as the various monthly schedules that can be utilized when taking HRT. Finally, helpful tips are given on how to adjust to HRT as well as on how to comfortably and safely discontinue HRT if you desire to do so.

History of HRT

The use of hormones after menopause is a recent innovation in human history. Relatively few women even survived the rigors of more primitive societies to face the issue of postmenopausal aging. How long a woman lived did not depend on sophisticated hormonal therapies synthesized in a laboratory but rather on a combination of good genes, familial longevity, a healthy lifestyle with adequate nutrition, balanced responses to stress and a balance of physical activity and rest. Only since the turn of the century have women begun to outlive their menopause and continue to do so for several decades.

Scientists first isolated estrogen and progesterone in the laboratory in their purified state during the 1920s. In the decades before this advance, physicians prescribed various formulations of the whole gland. Animal ovaries were powdered, pulverized and liquefied and then given by health care providers to women who had gone through surgical menopause or to those who suffered from menstrual cramps. Use of hormones remained limited throughout the 1930s and 1940s. By the 1950s and 1960s, the benefits of estrogen in treating menopausal symptoms were understood and appreciated and its use became widespread. A number of books and articles were written during this era about estrogen's many benefits, both real and fancied. Many women benefited from the relief estrogen brought from unpleasant hot flashes, vaginal dryness, mood swings and other symptoms. Women were told that estrogen would even enhance their attractiveness and youthfulness. However, very little was understood or communicated to women about the risks of using estrogen.

The first adverse reports about estrogen therapy surfaced in 1975. Several research studies published that year linked estrogen use in postmenopausal women with cancer of the lining of the uterus (also called the endometrium). In those studies women who used estrogen were four to eight times more likely to develop this cancer. Fearful of cancer, postmenopausal women avoided estrogen in dramatic numbers, and physicians were equally hesitant about prescribing it. This decline lasted for several years until further research studies showed that the combined use of estrogen and progestins (synthetic forms of progesterone) offered women excellent protection against the development of cancer of the uterine lining. In the regimens tested, women used estrogen 25 days each month, adding a progestin the last 10 to 14 days of the monthly treatment schedule.

Today, physicians prescribe estrogen and some form of synthetic or natural progesterone to combat early and postmenopausal symptoms. Physicians currently are able to use HRT with much greater wisdom and very little risk. Many research studies done on HRT now enable physicians to prescribe specific types of hormones and dosage regimens for each individual woman's needs. A 1994 Gallup Poll indicated that 40 percent of all menopausal women in the United States use HRT. This low percentage appears to be related to poor compliance, myths or fears about estrogen use, the wish to pass through menopause naturally, and lack of support for finding the right regimen for the individual woman.

Working with Your Physician

Steps to Follow Before Starting HRT

If you are considering beginning HRT therapy, scheddule an initial health evaluation to determine if any risk factors exist that the use of hormones could aggravate. In addition to determining the suitability of your using HRT, a good medical evaluation will identify any undiagnosed health issues that can then be adequately treated.

A pre-HRT evaluation may vary in its components depending on your medical status and what specific menopause-related health problems your physician is most concerned about. Tests used in evaluating a woman for HRT may include the following:

1. A complete physical examination, including a pelvic exam and a breast exam.

2. A PAP smear to determine a cancerous or precancerous lesion of the cervix.

3. Blood tests to check liver function, blood sugar, cholesterol, triglyceride, calcium and phosphorus levels, as well as tests of thyroid function.

4. Complete blood count to check for anemia, as well as a urinalysis.

5. Mammography and professional breast examination to check for breast cancer. Mammograms done by experienced radiologists are capable of detecting 90 percent of all breast cancers.

6. Bone density studies (dual x-ray absorptiometry, DEXA) to help determine the level of bone loss. This is an important test for women who may be at higher risk for osteoporosis.

7. A review of your family medical history to gather clues about your risk of cardiovascular disease, osteoporosis, and breast and other cancers.

8. Endometrial biopsy or vaginal ultrasound may be done to check for hyperplasia (overgrowth) of the uterine lining and endometrial cancer. A progesterone challenge test may also be done after menopause to check for endometrial hyperplasia.

If the results of these tests do not contraindicate the use of HRT and you decide to use hormonal therapy, expect frequent follow-up visits with your doctor. He or she will want to monitor the amount of hormones you are taking and their effect on menopausal symptoms, as well as your general health. Most physicians recommend annual visits. At this time, you should discuss any remaining symptoms or possible side effects that have developed since beginning HRT. Blood pressure will be monitored at each visit and a breast and pelvic exam done to check the health of these tissues. Most importantly, it is an excellent time to ask your doctor any questions that you may be concerned about. It is crucial that you tell your doctor any concerns or issues that you may have regarding your therapy. If you are not satisfied with your physician's answers or feel that your physician is standoffish or abrupt, you may wish to seek another opinion or doctor in your community. Unexpressed concerns that are not discussed with your physician may delay the diagnosis and treatment of health problems that can arise during the course of treatment. The best results occur when a true partnership exists between doctor and patient.

Estrogen Therapy

Estrogen is taken as a supplement to compensate for the lack of estrogen circulating through your body as your ovaries begin to age. A great deal of research has resulted in three forms of natural and synthetic estrogen that are synthesized in the laboratory (produced in our bodies as estradiol, estrone and estriol). Not only are different types of estrogen available, but they can be administered by different routes which allow for great flexibility. These three major types of estrogen are usually differentiated in clinical practice based on their routes of administration which include oral, transdermal and cream.

Oral Estrogen Tablets

Many women take estrogen by mouth in pill form, known as "oral estrogen." Estrogen tablets are the most commonly used form of ERT. The estrogen tablets available on the market in the United States are composed of different forms of estradiol and estrone. As you may remember, estradiol is the main type of estrogen manufactured by the ovaries, and estrone is the primary type of estrogen that we produce after menopause. Estriol, the weakest and probably safest type of natural estrogen, is not available as replacement therapy in the United States, although it is available in Canada and Europe.

The most commonly prescribed estrogen tablet is Premarin (Wyeth-Ayerst Laboratories), a conjugated equine estrogen derived from a pregnant mare's urine. It has been available since 1941, and much of the medical research has been done using this product. As a result, the benefits and side effects of Premarin are very well understood. Another benefit of Premarin is that it comes in a wider variety of doses than any of the other estrogen products. This allows for much more flexibility in determining the optimal treatment dosage for each woman user. Besides Premarin, currently available are generic, conjugated estrogen and synthetic and semisynthetic estrogen compounds. Other products include Ogen (Abbot), which contains estrone, and Estrace (Meade-Johnson), which contains estradiol.

Women should avoid using nonsteroidal synthetic estrogens. One of these drugs, called diethylstilbestrol (DES), was used several decades ago to prevent miscarriage in women with high-risk pregnancies. Unfortunately, many female children of these women have subsequently developed vaginal and cervical abnormalities including cancer. Most doctors also avoid estrogen tablets combined with a tranquilizer such as Menrium (Roche). Librium, the medication used to help treat mood problems in this particular formulation, is habit forming and can cause drowsiness. Because estrogen is used on an almost daily basis, the addition of tranquilizers can produce undesirable side-effects with long-term use.

The use of estrogen in pill form has some drawbacks. In the traditional regimen, women use estrogen 25 days per month with one week off (much like the birth-control pill). During this "off" time, some women find that their menopausal symptoms, such as hot flashes, recur. Other women dislike having to track pill intake. These two problems can be remedied by placing the woman on continuous therapy, where she is taking estrogen every day of the month. Obviously, women who dislike having to take a tablet each day would do better switching to another route of administration.

A more serious drawback to the use of oral estrogen is that after ingestion, a large amount of estrogen is concentrated in the digestive tract. When estrogen passes through the intestinal tract, intestinal bacteria transform the estrogen chemically. This can change the type as well as the potency of the estrogen that is reabsorbed back into the body. Once the estrogen is reabsorbed, it enters the blood circulation and is transported to the liver. In the liver, estrogen is again metabolized and converted to the other forms before it finally enters the general circulation. How efficiently this occurs depends on the health of the liver. Many nutritional factors such as fat, sugar, alcohol and B-complex vitamin intake affect liver function, as does pre-existing liver disease. Women with a history of liver or gallbladder disease or hypertension and clotting problems (which are affected by various actions in the liver) may do well to avoid oral estrogen. They might instead use another route that circumvents the digestive tract and instead, disperses estrogen into the general circulation.

For those women who can assimilate oral estrogen without a problem, the most commonly prescribed dose of Premarin is 0.625 mg. However, some women need higher doses such as 0.9 mg or 1.25 mg to attain symptom relief. Occasionally, women drop their doses in half to 0.3 mg to avoid side effects, but this dose may not be enough to benefit bones and avoid bone loss. Only trial and error will tell you which dose works best for you. Women who have already had a hysterectomy can take estrogen tablets alone because they obviously have no risk of developing uterine cancer. Women who have an intact uterus should always take a formulation that includes progestin for at least 10 to 13 days of each month for cancer protection.

Transdermal Estrogen

The transdermal system, marketed under the name Estraderm (IBA Pharmaceuticals), was created to avoid the problems inherent in oral estrogen's first pass through the liver. In this innovative system, estrogen is absorbed into the general circulation through a medicated patch on the skin. This method avoids the initial pass through the digestive tract and liver, so women with liver and gallbladder disease are more likely to be able to tolerate ERT. This is also true for women with hypertension and clotting problems, provided clotting factors are normal.

Another benefit is that the patch dispenses estrogen continuously, rather than in one large burst like the tablet. The delivery of estrogen into the body throughout the day and night more closely resembles your body's own estrogen production. Because the body is receiving estrogen on a continuous basis, a woman is less likely to suffer from symptoms which can occur with estrogen pill when hormones are stopped for a week each month.

What does the patch look like? Many women compare it with a small, round, clear Band-Aid that is several inches in size. It is placed on the skin of the abdomen, buttocks or thigh and changed twice a week. Each patch contains a reservoir of estrogen placed in a membrane that releases estrogen at a controlled, standardized level. The nonabsorbent patch allows for greater freedom because it can be kept on while you shower or bathe.

Unlike the estrogen pill, there is not as much flexibility of dosage range. Basically, the transdermal patch is available in two dosages: 0.05 mg and 0.1 mg. Some women find they do not tolerate these dosages well and develop side effects. To decrease the amount of hormone released from the patch, part of the backing can be occluded by a small piece of ordinary adhesive bandage. This reduces the total surface area of the skin exposed to the hormone. Some women prefer to use oral estrogen because it is less expensive than the patch. Finally, ten percent of all patch users develop skin irritation from the patch's adhesive. To reduce the likelihood and severity of the skin reaction, apply the patch on different areas of your skin. The buttocks area seems to tolerate the patch best. Be sure to wait at least a week before reusing a prior site. During times of acute irritation, you can change the patch more frequently, every 12 to 24 hours; if needed, talk to your doctor about ways to relieve skin irritation. You may also want to remove the patch before swimming or soaking in a hot tub and reapply it once you have dried your skin.

As with oral estrogen, the patch is used in conjunction with progesterone if the woman still has an intact uterus, and progesterone should be taken for the recommended number of days each month. The patch appears to be as effective in relieving menopausal symptoms as the oral estrogen tablets. Studies to date suggest that its effect on calcium absorption and blood lipids are almost identical to oral estrogen.

Estrogen Vaginal Cream

The use of estrogen vaginal cream is much more limited in its clinical applications. Estrogen cream is primarily applied to the vagina and urethral area to prevent atrophy and breakdown of the tissues caused by lack of natural estrogen. Though estrogen is absorbed from the vaginal mucosa into the bloodstream and can affect other parts of the body, the effects tend to be undependable. Occasionally, however, my patients complain of more generalized side effects from using the vaginal cream, such as breast tenderness or mild fluid retention. These side effects often occur early in the course of treatment. Because of the vaginal atrophy that exists when women first begin treatment, estrogen tends to be absorbed rapidly. This can cause the blood levels of estrogen to rise significantly. However, once the estrogen thickens the vaginal walls and changes the cellular pattern of the mucous membranes to a more youthful and healthier condition, estrogen absorption into the bloodstream slows down. (It may or may not restore lubrication; the use of a lubricant cream or gel may still be needed.) Not only will estrogen thicken the vaginal wall, making it less traumatized by sexual inter-course or foreplay, but it also reduces the incidence of bladder infections.

Another benefit of the vaginal cream is that, like the transdermal patch, it does not make an initial pass through the liver. As a result, the use of estrogen vaginal cream may not aggravate liver or gallbladder disease, hypertension or clotting tendencies, unless clotting factors are abnormal. However, women with pre-existing breast cancer or who are also positive for estrogen receptors may not be good candidates for estrogen vaginal creams. This is currently being debated and the contro-versy may be resolved by using small topical doses with low risk.

Premarin cream is one of the most commonly used vaginal creams, although other brands are available. Premarin cream comes with an applicator that allows for the use of two to four grams per day (as calibrated by the applicator). One-half to one full applicator of Premarin cream will delivery 1.25 to 2.5 mg of estrogen to the vaginal tissues. Many women find, however, that they function quite well at smaller doses, often as little as one-eighth of an applicator.

Initially, you may want to use estrogen cream daily, at least for the first week or two. Be sure that the most sore or abraded areas come directly in contact with the cream, either through placement of the applicator or by applying the cream to sore and tender areas with your fingers. After healing has begun and sexual activity is more comfortable, many women reduce usage to two or three times per week. Use it as often as required to keep your vaginal tissues healthy and functional.

Vaginal cream has several drawbacks, none of which are serious. The creams tend to be messy and can leak into your underwear. Estrogen vaginal cream should not be used as a lubricant or applied prior to lovemaking. Some men are con-cerned about the adverse effects of absorbing estrogen through their penis if the cream is still in the woman's vagina during sex-ual activity. Estrogen cream can, however, be inserted following lovemaking, particularly just prior to retiring at night.

If you are concerned about using estrogen for protection against osteoporosis or cardiovascular disease, estrogen vaginal cream is inadequate to meet these goals. You will have to use additional estrogen, either by the transdermal or oral routes to keep your blood levels of estrogen consistently high enough to confer protection. In addition, a course of progesterone needs to be used, at least every three months, to "clean out" the uterus and allow the lining to shed. The addition of progesterone will help mature the lining of the uterus and thereby prevent the buildup of cells that can lead to hyperplasia or even cancer.

Rarely, androgen cream is also prescribed in very small dosages, usually in 1 or 2 percent concentration, to help prevent vaginal discomfort and soreness. It is also used to help restore sexual desire or libido, a fairly common problem in menopausal women. It has certainly been an issue for many of my patients because it affects their quality of life, as well as the pleasurable aspect of their intimate relationships. Like estrogen cream, androgen cream is applied daily for a week or two and then decreased to twice-weekly applications. Care must be taken not to overdose, since masculinization side effects such as excessive hair growth or clitoral enlargement can occur.

Alternative Routes for Estrogen Administration

You may also hear of several other routes of estrogen delivery. These methods tend to be used rarely or are more readily available in other countries.

Intramuscular Injection. Intramuscular injection was used occasionally before the development of the transdermal patch and may still be used for women who can neither take oral estrogen nor the transdermal patch. This method does have several disadvantages. The injection delivers large amounts of estrogen directly into the bloodstream, then diminishes to lower levels with time. Thus, there is not a continuous delivery of the hormone to the body that the transdermal patch now makes possible. Finally, injections are usually given at monthly intervals and require administration in a physician's office which are expensive in terms of time and money.

Subcutaneous Pellets. A subcutaneous pellet of estrogen therapy, used during the 1960s and 1970s, is not currently a method of treatment. The hormone was impregnated into a solid pellet which was then implanted by a small incision into the subcutaneous fat of the buttocks or abdomen. The pellets would dissolve slowly, releasing hormone into the fatty tissues. Research is now oriented toward trying to improve types of implants, as well as the more controlled release of the hormone into the system. Thus, it is possible that subcutaneous implants will be used once again for ERT.

Buccal Estrogen. A low-dose estrogen tablet has been developed that can be placed directly against the mucous membranes inside the mouth. The tablet dissolves rapidly and the estrogen that is released from the tablet is absorbed directly into the bloodstream. Estrogen released by this method is sufficient to relieve common symptoms such as hot flashes. It is still pending approval by the US Food and Drug Administration.

Estrogel. Estrogel is a form of estrogen replacement therapy used frequently in France. The estrogen is in a gel-base that is rubbed on the skin of the abdomen and absorbed into the body. The dose can be varied easily by changing the amount of gel used.

Progesterone Therapy

Before the 1980s, all progesterone therapy had to be administered by injection. Women who required progesterone treatments for specific medical problems had to go to the doctor's office for every treatment. The development of oral progesterones made this hormone more readily available. Initially, progesterone was combined with estrogen in birth-control pills for younger women. Progesterone's important role in preventing endometrial cancer in postmenopausal women on ERT was discovered in the 1970s. It rapidly became part of the standard hormonal regimen for postmenopausal women who still had their uterus intact. The traditional form of treatment does not, however, use the same natural form of progesterone produced by your ovaries. Instead, a synthetic form called a progestin is used. It was not until recently that some physicians actually began to use natural progesterone for postmenopausal support. In this section, I will discuss both the synthetic and natural forms of progesterone.

Oral Progestins. Oral tablets of synthetic progesterone are the most widely prescribed form of progesterone. The progestins change the cells of the uterine lining from a pattern of rapid growth to a more mature form. The cells become secretory in nature, which prepares the uterus to nourish and maintain an early pregnancy during the active reproductive years. With the proper dose and ratio to estrogen, once a woman stops progesterone the uterine lining is sloughed off and a menstrual period or bleeding episodes occur. All of the accumulated proliferated cells, tissue and blood leave the body. No pile-up of abnormal cells occurs and the uterine lining is left healthy and ready for the next month's estrogen therapy, therefore reducing the risk of uterine cancer.

Reaching this beneficial goal requires only small doses of progestins, usually doses of 5 to 10 mg. Some women need slightly higher or lower doses. Women who develop side effects such as fatigue and depression may need to drop their dose to as low as 1.25 mg per day, while others must use up to 10 mg per day to achieve the best therapeutic effects.

Progestins can be used for other aspects of menopause in addition to their normal role in preventing uterine or endometrial cancer. For example, physicians often prescribe progestins for women transitioning into menopause who have excessive bleeding due to an imbalance of female hormones. Women may produce too much estrogen without ovulating. This causes heavy periods, which can last as long as 10 to 20 days, or even longer. Progestins taken for one week each month or for 10 to 12 days are usually effective in controlling this bleeding. They are also used during the early menopausal years when a woman is no longer bleeding. Progestins are given as a "challenge test" to see if the lining of the uterus is still being stimulated. If you bleed after stopping the progestins, your body is still producing estrogen. In this case, the progestins must be used on a monthly basis, even without additional estrogen therapy. The risk of endometrial cancer is higher in women taking no hormones than those on HRT because of a woman's unopposed endogenous estrogen.

The most commonly used brand of progestins is Provera (Upjohn). Norlutate (Parke-Davis) is also frequently prescribed, but it may cause side effects similar to androgens such as oily skin and acne. A third progestin currently on the market is Amen (Carnick).

Oral Micronized Progesterone. Synthetic progestins were used originally instead of natural progesterone because they may be taken orally. Unfortunately, natural progesterone cannot be ingested because it is destroyed during digestion and never reaches the bloodstream. In recent years, a new micronized form of progesterone is available that is protected from destruction by stomach acid and enzymes and can be absorbed and utilized by the body. Made from the natural progesterones found in yams and soybeans, oral micronized progesterone has gained wide acceptance by physicians as a treatment for premenstrual syndrome (PMS). I began to prescribe natural progesterone over a decade ago to my PMS patients and I am very pleased by the response to this treatment. It seems to be particularly helpful in controlling the emotional symptoms of PMS such as anxiety and mood swings.

Menopausal women are beginning to use this form of progesterone more frequently because it causes fewer side effects than the synthetic progestins. While the progestins can cause depression, fatigue, bloating, breast tenderness, and also adversely affect blood cholesterol levels, the natural progesterone seems to cause fewer adverse reactions. However, natural progesterone may still cause drowsiness because of its sedative effect on the brain.

The main drawback to natural progesterone is its expense. It is more expensive than the synthetic progestins, a deterrent for women on a tight budget. In menopausal women, dosages of 200 mg daily can be effective, although the dose can vary in either direction. Like the synthetic progestins, it is used 10 to 13 days per month and appears to confer an equal amount of protection against uterine cancer. Besides the oral form, it can also be obtained as a rectal or vaginal suppository. PMS patients use this route of administration successfully, as vaginal suppositories allow excellent local intake of progesterone into the uterus. Ask your physician about natural progesterone if it seems like it might be the right form of progesterone for you.

Progesterone Skin Cream. Pro-Gest®Cream is applied to the skin and absorbed into the general circulation. It is a natural progesterone derived from the barbasco plant, a giant yam that grows in the jungles of Mexico. It is also extracted from other plants grown in Europe and Asia. Because it is absorbed through the skin, it bypasses the liver, thereby escaping liver metabolism. Unlike the synthetic progestins, there are few side effects reported by its use.

Pro-Gest cream is applied to the skin twice daily in one-quarter to one-half teaspoon amounts. It is generally used on rising and before going to bed at night. It can be applied to any area of your skin. Many women will rub it into their chest, abdomen, arms or back. If the cream is absorbed rapidly (under two minutes), it means that the body needs a higher dose and a slightly higher amount may be used. Few physicians have any experience using Pro-Gest cream to date and it is more likely to be used by physicians knowledgeable about alternative therapies. You may want to check with physicians practicing alternative therapies in your area to find one prescribing progesterone topical cream.

General Guidelines of Hormonal Use

Understand and follow these principles if you wish to obtain the best results from HRT. These relate to dosage, route of administration, regimen and frequency, choice of physician, and proper cessation.

Choose the Lowest Dose That Works

In general, use the lowest possible dosage of both estrogen and progesterone that will relieve your symptoms and prevent long-term health problems associated with hormonal deficiency such as osteoporosis and cardiovascular disease. Medical research has shown this to be 0.625 mg for the Premarin oral tablet and 0.05 mg for the estrogen transdermal patch. If you start at higher doses, you are more likely to encounter side effects such as anxiety, mood swings, fluid retention and breast tenderness. Many women who could benefit from HRT discontinue it because of unpleasant (and often unnecessary) side effects.

Some women find that even the tiniest dosage of estrogen normally prescribed, 0.3 mg, provides adequate symptom relief. However, such a low dosage may not provide sufficient protection against the development of bone loss or cardiovascular disease. Thus, women with high risk factors for developing either problem should not use this minimal dosage. To know your risk potential, have your physician perform the appropriate tests. If you feel comfortable at the smaller dosages, you may wish to combine estrogen with the alternative therapies described later in this book. At the other end of the spectrum, you may feel your best only when using estrogen in the high-dose ranges. If you have experienced a surgical menopause below the age of 40, you may need more estrogen than women who go through natural menopause at a later age. Obviously, with estrogen, one dosage does not fit all women and therapy must be carefully individualized to each woman's needs.

Progesterone should also be used in the lowest possible dose to prevent side effects. This is particularly true for the synthetic progestins, which can cause the most problems. As mentioned earlier, I have had patients drop their dosages to as low as 1.25 mg to avoid common progestin-induced side effects such as fatigue, depression and bloating. I've also seen physicians increase the dosage to as high as 15 to 20 mg per day on a short-term basis to stop heavy menstrual bleeding in a woman transitioning into menopause. Your physician will order the lowest dose to confer protection against uterine cancer, yet one that is comfortable for you. This may require some fine tuning and tests such as a vaginal ultrasound under the guidance of your physician.

Choose The Route of Administration That Is Most Comfortable

Some women find it difficult to remember to take one or two pills each day. They may occasionally miss days. This does not create the same potential problem that missing a day or two of birth control pills will, because menopausal women do not have to worry about unplanned pregnancies (unless they are in the early stages of menopause). However, if you find pill-taking too challenging or unpleasant, then you are better off asking your physician about the alternative routes of administration such as the estrogen transdermal patch or progesterone cream.

Choose the HRT Regimen That Suits You Best

Traditionally, estrogen was taken only three weeks per month with one week off. Provera, a common progestin, was added during the last 10 to 13 days of the regimen to prevent the development of endometrial cancer. Taking one week off estrogen each month reduces the time during which the uterine lining is exposed to estrogen, therefore, reducing the risk.

However, some women find that menopausal symptoms such as hot flashes recur during this "off" week. In addition, many women dislike the bleeding, similar to a regular menstrual period, that occurs within a few days after the hormones are stopped. Even though the bleeding tends to be lighter and even diminishes or stops over time, many women find it an annoyance. While some physicians still use the traditional three weeks on, one week off regimen with their patients, other regimens have become very popular in recent years. With one protocol, estrogen is taken every day and a progestin is added on an intermittent basis, usually during the first 12 days of the calendar month. More than two-thirds of the women on this regimen, if they have a uterus, experience bleeding when administration of progestin stops after day 12. With combined continuous therapy, both estrogen and low doses of progestins are used on a daily basis without stopping. Women on this regimen may experience irregular bleeding during the first six months of treatment, which then diminishes. With both continuous and combined continuous therapy regimens, bleeding often doesn't persist indefinitely. For many women, bleeding becomes lighter and stops entirely after a few years. This occurs as the endometrium eventually becomes inactive.

Both these regimens appear to protect women against the development of uterine cancer as well as does the "on-off regimen." Also, constant daily hormonal intake protects women better from recurrence of menopausal symptoms.

Pick a Physician Who Will Tailor HRT to Your Needs

One of the most important factors in developing a successful menopause relief program is to work with a physician who is knowledgeable and dedicated to helping you achieve the best therapeutic results. How does one find such a physician? You might try asking your friends for a referral. Choose several physicians and interview them to determine if their philosophy of HRT and personality fit with you. Ask many questions and evaluate the responses. Remember, this relationship between you and your physician will be a long-term one.

Attaining the goal of the best HRT regimen for you may require considerable tinkering over time with both dosages and formulations until the right results are achieved. Though some women adapt easily and effortlessly to their hormonal regimen, others need the expertise and help of an empathetic physician to achieve the results they desire. However, if you have made the decision to use HRT and believe strongly that these hormones can provide you with real benefits, it is worth the time and persistence. The benefits that HRT can provide are discussed in detail in the following chapters.

Stop Hormone Use Gradually

What if you've been on HRT for some time and now feel that it's time to stop using it? While many women stay on HRT indefinitely, other women do not feel the need to continue with HRT after using it for a short period of time. Once the initial symptoms are relieved and the body is adjusted to the postmenopausal period, they may wish to see how they feel without hormones. Others dislike the side effects that develop with HRT, so choose to discontinue it. Whatever the reason for stopping HRT, don't do it abruptly. This can cause a severe recurrence of symptoms (such as hot flashes) as your body reacts to the rapid decline in estrogen. Just as during the early postmenopausal period, the pituitary pumps out high levels of FSH in an attempt to make your body produce the estrogen that has suddenly disappeared. Hot flashes and night sweats can reappear as the pituitary-hypothalamic axis goes off balance.

Be sure to stop HRT use very slowly. I often recommend cutting the dose of estrogen by one-half each month for one or two months. Then cut back to every other day for a month, followed by twice a week for a month, and finally to once a week for a month. Continue to take your progesterone on your regular schedule until you have stopped the estrogen entirely, then discontinue it. If your symptoms recur in too uncomfortable a fashion, you can always begin HRT use again.

Using HRT in the safest and most comfortable dosage and regimen for your individual needs will provide the best therapeutic results with the least risks and side effects. What you can expect in terms of symptom relief from your HRT program is discussed in the next chapter.

Types of Estrogen

Oral estrogen tablets
Transdermal estrogen patch
Estrogen vaginal cream
Intramuscular injection
Subcutaneous pellets
Buccal estrogen
Estrogel

Types of Progesterone

Synthetic progestins
Oral micronized progesterone
Vaginal or rectal progesterone suppositories
Progesterone skin cream

Pros & Cons
of HRT

$\mathcal{T}$he question of whether or not to use HRT is a major issue for women who would like to try this therapy but have concerns about possible side effects or long-term risks of HRT. Because your protocol should be individualized to your own health profile and family history, the more informed you are about the pros and cons of hormone use, the better choices you will make.

Women vary greatly as to how appropriate HRT is for them. Many women are excellent candidates. They have menopausal symptoms that will benefit from treatment, without significant pre-existing health problems that may cause adverse reactions to the therapy. Other women find the decision is less clear cut. Some may experience side effects even more unpleasant than hot flashes and other menopausal symptoms. A few women have health problems that HRT will aggravate; others have a family history of a high-risk disease that makes HRT potentially dangerous.

Women must balance the potential benefits against the risks, understanding that no outcome is perfect. This quandary is faced by women who have severe hot flashes or accelerated bone loss, a strong family history of estrogen-dependent breast cancer, or large uterine fibroid tumors with a history of heavy bleeding. In such cases, there may be no easy answer. HRT use for a high-risk woman should include great care and close monitoring.

This chapter is divided into five sections. The benefits of ERT are discussed in the first section, the risks in section two. Health problems aggravated by ERT are covered in section three. The benefits and risks of progesterone therapy are presented in sections four and five. Use this information as a guide when discussing your questions about HRT with your physician as you work together developing a good treatment strategy.

Benefits of Estrogen Replacement Therapy (ERT)

Consider using ERT if you suffer from the following conditions or symptoms. Many of the conditions included in this section will be discussed in detail in later chapters.

Symptoms Decrease after Surgical Menopause

A surprising number of women under age 40 undergo hysterectomies for medical reasons. These problems include pelvic infections (an increasingly common problem), cancer, endometriosis, uterine fibroid tumors, severe bleeding and pain due to scar tissue. When the disease process is severe or widespread, the ovaries are removed along with the uterus. Usually surgeons will try to leave at least one ovary or part of an ovary, because the remaining ovary will continue to secrete hormones. When it is not possible and both ovaries are lost, the woman undergoes a sudden drop in hormone levels.

Unlike the gradual decrease in hormone levels that occurs with each advancing decade, this abrupt drop throws the woman's body into shock. Women report feeling hot flashes, fatigue, depression, a loss of libido and other symptoms after surgery. They are also at much greater risk for developing osteoporosis over time. For these women it is advisable to begin hormonal replacement therapy at the time of surgery. Some women elect to mimic the natural menopause reduction in hormones by decreasing hormonal doses in their forties and discontinuing hormones entirely in their fifties, while some women elect to stay on hormones indefinitely. Alternative therapies alone are often not sufficient to prevent menopausal symptoms from developing in these women.

Eliminates Hot Flashes and Night Sweats

Eighty-five percent of postmenopausal women in the United States suffer from hot flashes, night sweats and poor sleep quality. Estrogen is very effective in relieving these symptoms. Many women elect to use it at the time of menopause to increase their comfort and sense of well-being. Estrogen is not a cure, however, because the hot flashes may return when replacement therapy is discontinued—the ovaries are not revitalized or regenerated in any way by the estrogen therapy.

Decreases Vaginal Dryness, Soreness and Pain During Intercourse

The drop in estrogen levels with menopause causes the vaginal walls to become thin, dry and easily traumatized by friction. This makes intercourse uncomfortable or painful. Without the estrogen support, the vagina actually shrinks. Estrogen replacement therapy is very effective in building up the vaginal lining and improving lubrication and resistance to friction. With the use of estrogen replacement therapy, sexual intercourse becomes more enjoyable and comfortable. The use of ERT can also help prevent repeated vaginal and bladder infections.

Reduces Anxiety, Irritability, Mood Swings, Fatigue and Depression

The loss of sleep at night due to hot flashes and sweating, as well as the drop in hormonal levels, can cause mood changes. Both estrogen and progesterone affect brain chemistry.

Progesterone has a sedative effect, while estrogen acts as a mood stimulant. If these hormones are out of balance during the menopause transition or deficient during the postmenopausal years, emotions can go haywire. The use of ERT will help restore emotional equilibrium. Many menopausal women are concerned because they seem to forget small details such as names and places and misplace objects more easily. Estrogen helps improve short-term memory in these women. The beneficial effects that ERT has on mental functioning appears to be maintained on a longer term basis. Although more controlled research is required to validate findings, recent studies indicate that the use of ERT reduces the risk of developing Alzheimer's disease. In a study done at the University of California, researchers checked the histories of 9,000 women in a retirement community and found that those on ERT were 40 percent less likely to develop Alzheimer's or other dementias. In another study completed at the University of Southern California, researchers found that in 253 elderly women, of those diagnosed with Alzheimer's only 7 percent were on ERT, as opposed to 18 percent of the other women who were using ERT.

Improves Skin and Muscle Tone

ERT helps the skin remain younger looking because it helps return moisture to the skin. As a result, the skin looks and feels smoother, softer, and "plumper." The skin also stays thicker. In addition, ERT helps maintain tone and strength in your body's muscle tissue. Breasts remain tauter; the muscles of the pelvic floor maintain better tone. Women who don't use ERT may complain about their muscles "sagging."

Prevents or Treats Osteoporosis

A number of medical studies have clearly shown that estrogen therapy decreases calcium loss from the bones after menopause. Because the effects of osteoporosis are so devastating (including loss of bone strength, thinning of bones, increased number of fractures and poor healing of fractures), women at high risk of osteoporosis may want to consider estrogen therapy. Sections later in this book will deal with this subject in depth.

There is evidence that ERT reduces the incidence of rheumatoid arthritis. It may also help prevent arthritic pain in those women who have already developed this condition.

Prevents Heart Attacks

The use of ERT helps prevent the development of cardiovascular disease by decreasing the dangerous LDL cholesterol levels (implicated in heart attacks) while elevating the beneficial HDL cholesterol. In addition, ERT has a beneficial effect on the blood vessels themselves. It relaxes smooth muscle in the blood vessel walls, which improves circulation throughout the body and helps reduce blood pressure. The entire subject of heart disease and menopause is so important I devote a chapter to it later in the book.

Improves Longevity

ERT reduces the death rate of women dying from osteoporosis, heart attack and, perhaps, stroke. In fact, estrogen decreases the mortality rate from heart attacks by one-third. As a result, women on ERT can gain a four-year increase in life expectancy.

Side Effects of Estrogen Replacement Therapy (ERT)

Women using ERT may suffer from side effects of the therapy as well as aggravation of pre-existing health problems. Side effects include fluid retention, tender breasts and weight gain, all three of which may be related. The other most common side effects include withdrawal or irregular bleeding, bloating, headaches, nausea, anxiety, vaginal discharge and estrogen allergy.

Although estrogen is generally well tolerated, some women may find that they experience one or more of these side effects. When this occurs, the dosage and route of administration can be altered to minimize the effects of these uncomfortable symptoms.

Withdrawal Bleeding. Eighty to ninety percent of women on combined HRT therapy experience withdrawal bleeding when the three weeks on, one week off regimen is utilized. Fewer women experience bleeding on continuous therapy. However, irregular bleeding and spotting (called break-through bleeding) can occur during the first six to nine months until the uterine lining becomes inactive. Many women dislike these bleeding episodes and find them a nuisance after menopause.

Fluid Retention. Women on ERT may rapidly gain several pounds due to fluid retention. In fact, I have had a number of patients gain as much as 10 to 15 pounds. If this weight is due to hormonal therapy and dietary habits are unchanged, the weight can be very difficult to lose. I have seen figure-conscious women go off ERT simply to lose the unwanted bloat. It may, however, be difficult to differentiate fluid retention from the accumulation of excess fat poundage. Estrogen does encourage fat deposition in the body. Also, as we age, women tend to gain weight more easily due to slowing metabolism associated with aging of the body and less efficient burning of calories. Women may find that restricting salt intake, daily walking and even an occasional herbal diuretic will help combat this problem.

Lower Abdominal Bloating. Symptoms of abdominal fullness or bloating can occur during the first few months of estrogen therapy. It is similar to the PMS bloating that many younger women experience one to two weeks prior to the onset of their menstrual period. If this symptom persists, you may need to decrease your estrogen dose.

Headaches. Occasionally women beginning ERT will complain about recurring headaches. Women with a previous history of migraines seem to be more at risk. These headaches are probably due to the excessive fluid retention occurring throughout the body due to the estrogen therapy. If this condition happens to you, you can try two things to remedy the problem: you can lower your dose of estrogen or, if you are taking oral estrogen tablets, you can switch to the transdermal patch. If the headaches continue, consult a physician who specializes in treating headaches. This is especially true for women who need ERT to prevent other health problems such as osteoporosis and cardiovascular heart disease. You may also choose, with assistance from your physician, to use the alternative therapies for relief of menopausal symptoms.

Nausea. Women on ERT can develop nausea similar to that experienced when first starting birth control pills or during the early months of pregnancy. Often this symptom diminishes over time and seldom requires discontinuation of treatment, except by very susceptible women. Changes in estrogen dose or route of administration may work. Using the transdermal patch to avoid the digestive route may prove effective. Ginger is an herb that has been researched as an antinausea remedy; when taken as a tea or in capsule form, it may reduce the severity of symptoms.

Anxiety, Irritability, Moodiness. Some women find that estrogen triggers emotional symptoms similar to PMS. Some patients complain about being grouchy, irritable and more difficult to get along with. Personal relationships may suffer when this occurs. If you are experiencing these side effects, decrease the dose until reaching a level that does not produce as much emotional upset and turmoil. If need be, you can take a tiny dose of estrogen supplemented with estrogen-containing herbs or vitamin E. This formula tends to be milder in effect and can help smooth out moods while relieving estrogen-related anxiety and irritability. Diet and exercise can play an important role. Also, it is important to evaluate the balance of estrogen and progesterone. Finally, testosterone and thyroid hormones may help to resolve the negative emotional symptoms.

Vaginal Discharge. Estrogen replacement therapy can stimulate the vagina to secrete an overabundance of lubrication. This can create a constant and annoying vaginal discharge. Although this discharge does not cause the itching, burning and other symptoms seen with a vaginal infection, it may occasionally require the use of a small tampon or sanitary napkin.

Estrogen Allergy. Women who are allergic to estrogen may experience symptoms like rashes, itching or nasal congestion. Sometimes a brand change or dose reduction will relieve the symptoms. If symptoms are distressing, it may be necessary to reevaluate estrogen use, discover remedies that will control the untoward reaction or substitute natural substances.

Health Problems Affected by Estrogen

Estrogen should be used cautiously and may be contraindicated in women with certain pre-existing medical conditions. Estrogen use may also be discouraged for women with a strong family history of certain female-related cancers. These medical conditions include the following: cancer of the endometrium, estrogen-dependent breast cancer, liver and gallbladder disease, hypertension, blood clotting, diabetes, uterine fibroid tumors and endometriosis.

Previously Diagnosed or Suspected Cancer of the Uterus or Endometrium. Cancer of the uterus is estrogen-dependent. During the mid-1970s estrogen used alone as a treatment for menopausal symptoms was found to increase the number of cases of uterine cancer four to eight fold. Although estrogen itself does not cause cancer, it can cause hyperplasia (the buildup of cells of the uterine lining). In some women, hyperplasia can progress to cancer if estrogen used without progesterone is continued. Numerous significant research studies have led to the conclusion that the use of progesterone with estrogen therapy protects against the development of this cancer. However, to be effective progesterone must be used at least ten days. In a British study done in 1991, women who took estrogen alone or combined with less than ten days of progestins had more than double the risk of endometrial cancer than those who took progestins for ten or more days each month.

Some women are more naturally prone to uterine cancer than others. Women who are significantly overweight (by more than 30 pounds) are at a higher risk of uterine cancer because their fat cells produce an increased amount of estrogen. Physicians may advise these women not to use estrogen therapy but to use instead a 10-day course of progestins to induce bleeding and shedding of the lining of the uterus. A prior history of hypertension and diabetes also appears to increase the risk of developing this disease. If you have these risk factors or a strong family history of cancer, you may want to carefully consider the risks and benefits of using ERT.

Endometrial cancer is generally detected at an early stage because it causes abnormal bleeding. If this condition is suspected, an endometrial biopsy is performed (a procedure done in a physician's office in which a small sampling of cells from within the uterus is removed using a small curette and a suction device). Luckily, the incidence of this disease is very low, and it is very treatable by hysterectomy and other modalities. The cure rate is very high if identified at an early stage.

Previously Diagnosed or Suspected Estrogen-Dependent Breast Cancer.   Breast cancer is one of the most common cancers of women (estimates are that one out of nine women will develop it during her lifetime). Many women are understandably concerned about the connection between estrogen and cancer, a somewhat controversial issue in medicine.

The indications against ERT use are quite straightforward in women who have known breast cancer. Women who have a previously diagnosed estrogen-dependent breast cancer will normally not receive ERT. Though estrogen does not initiate cancer and is not a carcinogen, it can stimulate the growth of a cancer that is already there. Thus, the major concern is that ERT could help promote a recurrence of the disease. Physicians are very wary of exposing patients to this risk, no matter how severe their menopausal symptoms. Some breast cancer patients

Middlebury Community
Library

explore alternative therapies in an effort to relieve their hot flashes and other symptoms.

Not all breast cancers, however, are estrogen-dependent. This type of cancer tends to be more common in younger women who are in their active reproductive years. It is much less common in postmenopausal women, especially those women at least five years into menopause. Postmenopausal women are much more likely to develop a breast cancer that is not estrogen-dependent. Sensitive testing is currently available that can determine whether a breast cancer is receptor positive.

The issue about whether the use of ERT can increase the risk of developing breast cancer in women who have not had the disease is much less clear-cut. It is a certainty that the incidence of breast cancer has risen to a one-in-nine lifetime chance of developing cancer—double the risk women faced in 1960. One theory relates these numbers to exposure to pesticides (which, once in the body mimic the action of estrogen). Another theory suggests that older women undergoing hormone therapy, ages 60 to 66, increase their risk significantly. Thus, some studies done in the United States and abroad show no increase in risk, while others show a positive correlation. After sorting through the data, many experts believe that ERT does not increase the risk of breast cancer in the short term. However, after 10 to 15 years of use, ERT does appear to increase the risk (but not the mortality rate) of breast cancer by 20 to 30 percent. Alcohol intake of more than one ounce per day is also correlated with increased risk. Other risk factors include a high-fat diet (which can elevate estrogen levels in certain high-risk women), early puberty, late menopause, and never having been pregnant.

Women with a strong family history of breast cancer in close relatives such as a mother or sister may also want to avoid using ERT. If this is the case with you, you may elect to use ERT only on a short-term basis for relief of severe symptoms or weigh carefully the long-term health risks.

If you feel that you are at high risk of developing breast cancer, you may choose to avoid using ERT, as well as

Middlebury Community
Library

minimize your alcohol intake and eat a low fat, high-fiber diet. If your breasts are tender and lumpy, you may want to avoid caffeine. Several studies have implicated caffeine as increasing benign breast disease. In addition, be sure to do a breast examination on yourself each month. After menopause, the breasts become less dense and are actually easier to examine. Soft, movable lumps are usually the non-troublesome kind; however, a small hard mass is more likely to be cancerous. If you find a new lump, be sure to have your physician evaluate it immediately. Doctors routinely do a breast exam during an annual visit.

The National Cancer Institute recommends that women over age 50 have an annual mammogram. This is especially necessary if you have large or lumpy breasts, which can make self-examination more difficult. Mammograms given to women over age 50 were found to accurately detect 10 cancers for every 1,000 women. On this basis many physicians will have base-line mammograms done on their younger patients so that accurate diagnosis of breast masses can be done in later examinations. The new generation of mammography machines emit very low doses of radiation, so they do not themselves present much of a cancer risk. An experienced radiologist can detect by mammography 90 percent of all breast cancers. This is a particularly helpful technique when women have a small, early-stage cancer that cannot yet be detected by manual breast examination.

Liver and Gallbladder Disease. Women with active liver disease should avoid oral estrogen replacement therapy. The liver plays a key role in breaking down estrogen and other drugs in the body for safe elimination; a liver that is compromised due to alcohol abuse, hepatitis or other factors cannot perform this function effectively. Under these circumstances, estrogen levels may rise to high levels and become toxic. Luckily, the transdermal estrogen patch sends the hormone directly into the general circulation, bypassing the liver and intestinal tract. Women with liver disease can use the patches as a preferred route of administration. Women with liver disease who are suffering from symptoms of vaginal or bladder atrophy may wish to use estrogen vaginal cream, which also bypasses the liver.

The use of estrogen replacement therapy can also increase the risk of gallbladder disease in susceptible women. Research studies show that women on ERT have a 2.5 times greater risk of developing gallstones, which may require surgical removal. This increased risk occurs because estrogen increases the cholesterol function of bile which can predispose women towards gallstone formation. Women at risk for gallbladder disease include those who have a family history of the disease, are obese, eat a high-fat diet, have an elevated cholesterol level, or are diabetic. Women with a Native American ethnic background also run a high risk of gallbladder disease and may not choose to use estrogen replacement therapy.

If you are at high risk of developing gallbladder disease, you should probably avoid using oral ERT. Use of the estrogen skin patch may be preferable to oral estrogen if your menopausal symptoms are quite severe and require at least the short-term use of ERT because the first pass-through of estrogen through the liver and bile is avoided with the patch. It is also important to cut your fat intake while emphasizing a high-fiber, vegetarian-based diet, and bring your weight down if you are very overweight.

Hypertension. In one out of twenty women, the use of oral estrogen tablets elevates blood pressure. Estrogen causes the release from the kidney of two enzymes, renin and angiotension, which can cause blood pressure to rise. This risk appears to be diminished in women using the transdermal patch or vaginal cream.

Hypertension is an important risk factor for heart attacks and strokes, so a rise in blood pressure following the use of ERT must not be taken lightly. All women using estrogen should have their blood pressure carefully monitored. Particular care should be taken to follow women closely who have pre-existing borderline hypertension.

Rarely, a woman will have an idiosyncratic rejection to ERT. In such a case her blood pressure becomes elevated with the use of even small doses of ERT, so she may need to discontinue this program entirely. Luckily, this only happens infrequently.

Blood Clotting (Thrombophlebitis). Women with a history of thrombophlebitis may, after discussion with their physician, decide to avoid oral estrogen tablets because they tend to cause an increased susceptibility to forming clots. This is particularly true in women who are very overweight. If your menopausal symptoms are severe, your physician may choose to begin with a low dose of estrogen and then monitor your blood to see if there are any changes in the anti-clotting factors. The transdermal patch and vaginal cream present less risk in their use than oral estrogen. They are the preferred route of administration in women with a clotting history.

Among the general population of women on ERT, the use of estrogen does not appear to increase the risk of clotting problems. Menopausal women tend to use lower dosages of estrogen, so this may be a function of dosage. In contrast, women on the birth control pill do run a higher risk of thrombophlebitis. This is because contraceptive pills contain far higher doses of estrogen than is used for ERT.

If you do have a problem with previous blood clots, it is important that you avoid smoking cigarettes. Smoking constricts the blood vessels and reduces the anticlotting factors. It is also desirable to avoid a sedentary lifestyle and to diet to your optimal weight if you are very heavy.

Diabetes. The problem of diabetes and estrogen use is an issue for some diabetic women. The facts are as follows. The low doses of estrogen used in ERT do not affect carbohydrate metabolism except in rare cases. However, the higher doses of hormones contained in some birth control pills may cause changes in glucose levels. Generally, diabetic women can use

ERT safely, but blood sugar levels should be monitored carefully by their physician.

Uterine Fibroid Tumors. Fibroid tumors occur when there is excessive growth in the muscular tissue of the uterus. Fibroids can grow to very large sizes in some women, enlarging the uterus to a size seen in pregnancy. These growths are usually seen in women during their menstrual years and are stimulated by estrogen. They may expand in size with the use of estrogen-dominated birth control pills, in pregnancy, or in women who secrete high levels of estrogen naturally. Women transitioning into menopause may experience an increased incidence of fibroid growth.

Fibroids can cause excessive menstrual bleeding and pelvic discomfort to the point of necessitating a hysterectomy. Usually they shrink after menopause when estrogen levels decline. However, with estrogen replacement therapy they may not experience this shrinking process. It is therefore recommended that women with large fibroid tumors avoid ERT or closely monitor its use. If bleeding or other fibroid symptoms become a problem on estrogen therapy, its use may need to be discontinued.

Endometriosis. Endometriosis occurs when the uterine lining implants into organs and tissues of the pelvic cavity such as the ovaries, bowel, bladder and ligaments. Like the normal uterine lining, these implants are stimulated by estrogen and may bleed on a monthly basis. However, unlike the blood and tissue of the uterine lining, the endometrial implants cannot shed their surface buildup through a monthly menstrual period. Instead, the internal bleeding causes irritation, pain and scarring inside the pelvis. Often, this is treated by surgery and hormonal therapies.

Normally, endometriosis tends to decline with menopause as estrogen stimulation recedes. Rarely, however, ERT may restimulate the endometrial implants. This may require stopping ERT.

Benefits of Progesterone Therapy

Although progesterone is prescribed by gynecologists for other reasons than estrogen replacement therapy, it is still an important therapy for menopausal women. The major indications for use of progesterone are as follows: prevention of endometrial cancer, reduction of hot flashes and prevention or treatment of osteoporosis.

Prevents Endometrial Cancer. As discussed earlier, prevention of endometrial cancer is the primary reason why physicians prescribe progesterone. Without the addition of progesterone to an estrogen treatment regimen, the incidence of endometrial cancer increases four to eight fold in women with an intact uterus. The importance of progesterone therapy has been emphasized in a number of significant medical studies. In one study cited by Don Gambrell, Jr., M.D. in the *American Family Physician,* 5,563 postmenopausal women were followed for nine years. In women using estrogen alone, the incidence of endometrial cancer was 390.6 cases per 100,000 women per year. In contrast, with combined estrogen and progesterone therapy, the incidence was only 99 cases per 100,000 women per year. Not only does progesterone confer protection in women using HRT, but it actually appears to protect against the development of endometrial cancer in all postmenopausal women. In the same study, women using no HRT at all were at higher risk than those on progesterone because of their own endogenous estrogen. These women developed 245.5 cases per 100,000 women per year. Not only has the rate of cancer declined with the use of progesterone, but those women who develop it tend to do so at a later age.

Reduces Hot Flashes. Progesterone used alone can relieve hot flashes and other vasomotor symptoms in about 60 to 80 percent of the women who use this therapy. Between 15 and 20 percent of women who are transitioning into menopause experience hot flashes even while they're still having fairly regular menstrual periods. Often these women also experience the heavy bleeding, premenstrual tension and other symptoms that characterize this stage. Unfortunately, ERT cannot be used to suppress such hot flashes because many of these women have higher than normal levels of estrogen and often are not ovulating regularly. Thus, ERT used alone could intensify the pre-existing state of hormonal imbalance. Progesterone can also be used to relieve hot flashes in women who are clearly postmenopausal, but for varying reasons cannot use estrogen (such as estrogen allergy or large uterine fibroid tumors).

Prevents or Treats Osteoporosis. Although estrogen helps prevent osteoporosis by inhibiting calcium loss from the bone, the addition of progesterone helps decrease calcium loss even more effectively; it also promotes new bone formation. As a result, progesterone therapy actually increases bone mass. Progesterone may do this by acting directly on bone by binding with receptor sites. This has been shown in a number of good medical studies. In one study reported in the *British Medical Journal* in 1988, women using combined progesterone and estrogen therapy had a five to six percent increase in vertebral bone density per year (the percent gain was slightly greater in women on continuous therapy versus cyclical therapy). In another study by Leonard and Doble, published in 1990 in *The American Journal of Gynecological Health,* progesterone and estrogen used in combination increased the bone mineral content significantly, even in women starting the therapy after age 60. As a result, the addition of progesterone to ERT provides more complete as well as more effective treatment for osteoporosis than ERT alone.

Side Effects of Progesterone Therapy

Women using progesterone therapy may suffer a number of uncomfortable side effects. This is particularly true for women using the commonly prescribed progestins, the synthetic forms of progesterone such as Provera. The side effects include the following: depression and mood changes, breast tenderness and enlargement, increased appetite, adverse effect on blood lipids and headaches.

Depression and Mood Changes. Some women find that hormonal replacement therapy improves their mood tremendously, while others find that progestins cause depression and mood changes. Not surprisingly, mood changes also accompany use of the birth control pill which contains much higher levels of hormones. In fact, younger women are usually warned that mood changes can occur. If this happens, they are either changed to another birth control pill or are taken off oral contraceptives altogether. Sometimes the addition of a B vitamin complex containing at least 25 to 50 mg of B_6 alleviates moodiness. If not, consider trying the natural forms of progesterone or stop the progestin altogether (which would mean stopping ERT if you are using combined therapy to avoid the risk of endometrial cancer).

Breast Tenderness and Enlargement. The addition of a progestin to ERT may intensify breast pain and tenderness. The two hormones used in combination may cause fluid retention or vascular congestion within the breast tissue. This may cause the breasts to actually enlarge and become heavier. In some women, this may feel similar to the breast symptoms that they experienced premenstrually during their active reproductive years.

Often, these symptoms are only temporary and recede spontaneously after one to two months. If they persist, you may want to decrease your dose of progestin as well as make simple dietary changes. Reducing salt intake and limiting or avoiding caffeine-containing foods and beverages such as coffee, black tea, cola drinks and chocolate may help decrease symptoms. Vitamin E and vitamin B_6 may also help to relieve symptoms of breast pain. If none of these suggestions work and the pain is severe, you may have to abandon the use of progestins or try the natural form.

Increased Appetite. Both natural progesterone and progestins may increase your appetite through their effect on the blood sugar level. Progesterone causes carbohydrates to be metabolized rapidly, so women feel hungrier at shorter intervals. In addition to your main meals, you may find that you need several small snacks throughout the day when using progesterone. Obviously this isn't acceptable to some women who do not like the feeling of increased hunger or are concerned about their food intake.

Adverse Effect on Blood Lipids. Unlike estrogen, which alters blood fats in a beneficial way by increasing the protective HDL cholesterol and lowering the dangerous cholesterol implicated in heart attacks and strokes, progesterone adds to a woman's risk of these serious diseases. This has been found to be true in birth control pills that contain higher dosages of progestins. Although these original contraceptive pills may have lowered the levels of HDLs, the newer progestins do not. Two recent studies published in *Lancet* in 1990 and the *American Journal of Medicine* in 1991 found no lowering of the HDL levels (in contrast to three studies published ten years previously). One of these studies used oral synthetic progestins and the other transdermal synthetic progestins.

Provera, the form of progesterone used for HRT in most women, does not appear to exert this negative effect on the HDL levels, especially in the small dosages used. In several studies done on women using combined estrogen and progestins for longer than a 12-month period, no adverse effect was seen on the blood lipid pattern due to progestin use. In fact, a recent study completed in 1993 by A. A. Nabulsi presented convincing data that HRT greatly decreases the risk of heart disease.

Headaches. Some women experience the sudden onset of migraine headaches with the use of progestins. This can occur particularly when first starting the medication. Progesterone can cause constriction of the blood vessels, which may trigger the headaches. (In contrast, estrogen causes relaxation and dilation of the blood vessel walls.)

In summary, carefully review the pros and cons of HRT use that I have discussed in this chapter. Be sure to discuss with your own physician any concerns you have about the benefits or side effects of using hormones. This will enable you and your physician to put together the most effective treatment plan with the least likelihood of adverse health effects.

Benefits of ERT

- Symptoms decrease after surgical menopause
- Eliminates hot flashes and sweating
- Decreases vaginal dryness, soreness and
     pain during intercourse
- Reduces anxiety, irritability, mood swings,
     fatigue and depression
- Improves short-term memory
- Improves skin and muscle tone
- Prevents or treats osteoporosis
- Prevents heart attacks
- Improves longevity

Side Effects of ERT

- Withdrawal bleeding
- Fluid retention
- Lower abdominal bloating
- Headaches
- Nausea
- Anxiety, irritability, moodiness
- Vaginal discharge
- Estrogen allergy

Health Problems Affected by ERT

- Cancer of the uterus or endometrium
- Estrogen-dependent breast cancer
- Liver and gallbladder disease
- Hypertension
- Blood clotting
- Diabetes
- Uterine fibroid tumors
- Endometriosis

Benefits of Progesterone

- Prevents endometrial cancer
- Reduces hot flashes
- Prevents or treats osteoporosis

Side Effects of Progesterone

- Depression and mood changes
- Breast tenderness and enlargement
- Increased appetite
- Adverse effects on blood lipids
- Headaches

4

Heavy, Irregular Bleeding & Hormonal Therapy

$\mathcal{M}$any women making the transition toward menopause notice changes in both the length of their menstrual cycle
and the amount of blood lost with each menstrual period. Often,
this occurs during the mid- to late-forties, although age can vary
greatly. Women can begin this process as young as their thirties
and as late as their late-fifties; it can last as briefly as one year or
as long as five or six years.

What Happens During the Transition

In the early stage of menopause, the follicles begin to
atrophy, reducing the ability to produce estrogen. Women ovu-
late less frequently, thereby producing less progesterone, or no
progesterone at all during certain months. In an attempt to force
the ovaries to manufacture more hormones, the levels of the pituitary hormone FSH become elevated. This is the hormone that
triggers follicular function in the ovaries. Paradoxically, the
ovaries may go into overdrive in response to the pituitary stimulation. In fact, for a time the ovaries may even produce high levels
of estrogen until they are finally exhausted. (When this occurs,
estrogen levels may drop permanently and menstruation ceases.)

As a result, hormonal levels may fluctuate during this time, and the balance between estrogen and progesterone is disrupted.

Although both estrogen and progesterone stimulation are needed for healthy menstruation, the overabundance of estrogen and lack of progesterone can cause changes in the menstrual cycle. Too much estrogen causes the uterine lining to grow and thicken excessively. Without the addition of progesterone during the second half of the cycle, the lining continues to thicken and proliferate until it finally outgrows its blood supply and begins to shed. Heavy, irregular bleeding can be the unfortunate result for many women.

The overabundance of estrogen or the imbalance of estrogen and progesterone may also trigger other problems during menopause. Many women complain of intense PMS symptoms, including mood changes, anxiety, irritability, depression and fatigue. Bloating, breast tenderness and food craving are also experienced frequently. Many of my patients say their personal relationships suffer as they go through the transition. Women may be more easily angered or more irritable with family and friends during the week or two preceding menstruation. Even their job performance can suffer because some women find it more difficult to concentrate or feel more "spaced out" during this time.

High levels of estrogen can stimulate the growth of uterine fibroid tumors. Fibroids, also called myomas, are benign growths of muscle and connective tissue, usually found in the wall of the uterus. This condition affects 40 percent of women over age 40. For many women, fibroids do not create a problem because the tumors are usually small and don't cause any symptoms. However, for some women in their thirties and forties, fibroids can become a real problem. In these women, the fibroids either grow to be so large or become so numerous that they put pressure on the bowel or bladder wall, causing discomfort, frequent urination, and changes in bowel habits. At times, the fibroids grow to be so large that a woman feels them in her uterus through the abdominal wall, and she can appear to be four to five months pregnant. Sometimes fibroids outgrow their blood supply, causing considerable discomfort. Fibroids can also cause heavy menstrual bleeding which can lead to anemia. In fact, the combination of bleeding due to hormonal imbalance and fibroid tumors along with PMS symptoms is so common during the menopausal transition these are called "garden variety" complaints.

Variations in Bleeding Patterns

When the menstrual period changes for most women during the transition, many variations in patterns can occur. Some lucky women simply begin to skip periods, with the interval between gradually increasing until they cease menstruating entirely. Often bleeding becomes lighter as periods occur less frequently. Other women have the opposite pattern; they experience heavy menstrual bleeding, often with a significant amount of blood lost each month. This can occur either in a rapid, heavy flow or in a more moderate flow over an unusually long period of time. Blood loss is not always limited to the duration of the menstrual cycle; some women spot between periods. Spotting also occasionally happens at midcycle as an accompaniment to "mittelschmerz," a slight pain that may occur at ovulation.

Heavy, profuse menstrual bleeding can be an uncomfortable experience. A 7- to 10-day menstrual period is fairly common. Often patients report unpredictable cycles, sometimes coming twice a month, and in some extreme cases lasting as long as 60 days. Women may need to use double pads or a pad and a tampon and change them frequently, as often as every hour or two in severe cases. Many times, even frequent changes of pads and tampons do not soak up all the blood loss. Profuse menstrual flow can also be accompanied by large blood clots, which can be painful to pass and may leave a woman feeling weak, fatigued, and fully drained of energy for a day or two each month. If this process is allowed to go untreated, the excessive blood loss over time can lead to anemia. Luckily, the heavy and irregular bleeding finally runs its course. In the final phase of menopause, the periods begin to occur at longer intervals and the bleeding slows down until menstruation finally ceases altogether.

Diagnosis of an Abnormal Bleeding Pattern

Heavy, irregular bleeding is very common during the transition, and it must be carefully evaluated by your physician. Although the heavy flow is usually due to hormonal imbalance, it can also be the result of uterine fibroids, polyps, or even uterine or cervical cancer. Although the likelihood is small, these problems need to be diagnosed early so that they can be cured.

All women with bleeding problems need a careful medical history and physical examination, including a pelvic exam, performed. Usually, a physician will have a complete blood count done to see if the patient is anemic. A PAP smear will help rule out cervical cancer and can even pick up many cases of endometrial cancer. However, the most accurate test that your physician can perform to diagnose the cause of bleeding is an endometrial biopsy. In this test, a thin pipette curette removes a sample of the uterine lining. This test can be done easily in a doctor's office. The cells are then examined under the microscope to look for any abnormalities that suggest hyperplasia or cancer.

Occasionally, doctors perform a more extensive diagnostic procedure called a dilation and curettage (D&C), particularly if the patient is experiencing heavy bleeding or polyps are suspected. The D&C requires anesthesia because the physician uses a scraping or suction technique to remove the lining of the uterus. Not only does this allow for the diagnosis of the problem through cell analysis, but the D&C also effectively stops the bleeding, at least temporarily.

Doctors may also request an imaging technique called an ultrasound. Ultrasound can be used to visualize the size and shape of any pelvic masses such as fibroid tumors that could be causing the bleeding. It can also be used to assess the thickness of the uterine lining to diagnose hyperplasia. Once the cause of the bleeding is accurately pinpointed, the proper treatment can be prescribed by your physician.

Treatment for Heavy, Irregular Flow

Unfortunately, if you are experiencing a heavy, irregular flow, you are not a good candidate for HRT. This is because your body is producing hormones erratically, often manufacturing huge amounts of estrogen. Although you are still having periods and bleeding profusely, there is plenty of estrogenic stimulation. What women don't need during this period is more estrogen.

If you are not ovulating regularly and your progesterone levels are most likely inadequate, progesterone therapy may be the ideal treatment to help you get through this rocky period. In fact, progesterone—usually the synthetic progestin, Provera—is the most effective medical treatment available for women in menopause transition. Progesterone is usually prescribed alone for one week or 10 to 12 days a month. It is usually taken in doses ranging from 5 to 10 mg per day.

Progesterone helps prevent the erratic heavy periods that distress many women. It will also help prevent the heavy buildup of endometrial lining by making sure that the lining is completely shed each month. By promoting a regular menstrual period each month, the use of progesterone can also help reduce the number of endometrial biopsies your physician needs to perform. Eventually estrogen levels will diminish to the point that menstruation no longer occurs. At this point, regular HRT can start.

A few physicians will also prescribe natural progesterone. This is available as a skin cream or in oral micronized progesterone tablets. Natural progesterone, like the synthetic forms, can be used to oppose the high estrogen levels present at this time. The cream can be rubbed directly into the skin in areas like the abdomen, while the tablets are taken by mouth. It may be difficult to find a physician in your area who has sufficient experience with these forms of progesterone. However, it might be worth exploring if you find that you do not tolerate the synthetic progestins well.

Low-dose birth control pills are also occasionally prescribed for women in transition. The FDA now considers low-dose birth control pills safe for use by women up to age 50, providing they are nonsmokers and do not have a history of blood clotting problems, gallbladder disease or hypertension. There are benefits to this therapeutic approach. The low-dose pills shut down your system, replacing the high and erratic levels of hormones your body is producing with a premeasured outside source. This helps control heavy, irregular bleeding and may decrease PMS symptoms in some women. It also confers protection against unwanted pregnancy as women enter midlife.

If the birth-control pill is well matched to your body's needs, your symptoms may smooth out and disappear. Unfortunately, many women can't tolerate the low-dose birth control pills. PMS-like symptoms may worsen, such as mood swings, bloating and cramps. These formulations do contain a synthetic estrogen that is much stronger than the "natural" estrogen used in HRT, such as Premarin. As a result, women on low-dose birth control pills may have an increased risk of having a stroke, developing hypertension or a blood-clotting problem. However, if you have had a good experience using birth-control pills in the past, you may want to explore this option.

For most women, one of these treatment options will work. Whether you decide to use synthetic progestins, natural progesterone, or a low-dose birth control pill, excessive bleeding problems can be controlled. You may need to try several dose regimens or forms of treatment if you encounter side effects. However, the decreased risk of anemia, hyperplasia, or even endometrial cancer that these treatments provide is well worth the time spent finding a plan that is right for you.

5

Hot Flashes & HRT

$\mathcal{H}$ot flashes and other vasomotor symptoms are the most common complaints surrounding menopause. These symptoms refer to brief episodes of heat and perspiration that usually begin to occur as the menstrual periods cease. In fact, 80 percent of American women experience hot flashes, with 40 percent of these women having symptoms severe enough to seek medical care. This high prevalence of hot flashes is seen in menopausal women throughout the Western world including Canada and Europe.

Variations in Hot Flash Incidence

Interestingly enough, the pattern we see in the Western world is not duplicated in many other cultures. Far fewer Japanese and Indonesian women experience hot flashes, with an incidence of only 10 to 15 percent. Mayan women living in the Yucatan in Mexico do not experience hot flashes at all. Their only symptom as they move into menopause appears to be menstrual cycle irregularities. A number of interesting studies suggest that this difference in prevalence of hot flashes is probably due to dietary factors. Women in Asian, Mayan, African and other cultures consume much higher levels of estrogen-containing plant-based foods than women in Western societies. Thus, even though their own levels of estrogen diminish at menopause, women in these other societies receive significant hormonal support from their diet.

Women in our country who do not suffer from hot flashes tend to eat a more vegetarian-based diet high in plant estrogens. Also, women who carry excess body weight may have fewer problems with hot flashes. This is because women with a greater mass of fat cells can continue to produce a form of estrogen called estrone. Estrone is manufactured from a precursor hormone called androstenedione made by the adrenal glands. This additional source of estrogen can be significant enough to prevent hot flashes in heavier women, even after their main source of estrogen, estradiol, has diminished in output from the ovaries. Conversely, thin women who carry less body fat may suffer more intensely from hot flashes.

Although most women don't begin to have hot flashes until they have ceased menstruating, 15 to 20 percent of women suffer from hot flashes during transition when they are still having a menstrual cycle. In addition, women who have gone through an abrupt, surgical menopause with removal of ovaries and uterus have a higher incidence of hot flashes than do women who undergo natural menopause. If not started on HRT, women who have had surgical menopause can suffer from severe, frequent hot flashes.

Symptoms of Hot Flashes

Many women sense a hot flash beginning a few seconds before it starts. Most women describe the hot flash itself as a sudden and intense episode of warmth and heat. These episodes arrive unexpectedly, and the woman suddenly notices that she feels very warm. The hot flashes usually begin above the waist, especially on the chest, face and neck, and then radiate to other parts of the body. The blood vessels of the skin dilate when the hot flash is occurring, causing the skin to become pink and rosy colored.

The hot flashes are often accompanied by varying amounts of sweating—mild in some women and profuse in others. With more severe episodes, women may become so wet that they have to change their clothes or bed sheets. After the initial period of warmth, the sweat cools down the skin temperature, causing shivering. This temperature instability may be very uncomfortable for many women, causing them to alternately shed or add clothes. The temperature changes that women feel have been evaluated in research studies. These studies have found measurable changes in skin temperature just before the hot flash begins. In addition, there is a 10 to 15 percent increase in pulse rate.

The hot flash usually lasts from 30 seconds to 5 minutes. However, in extreme cases, patients report hot flashes lasting as long as an hour. Frequency also varies. Some notice them infrequently, having only a few a year or once or twice a month. Many women will have hot flashes on a daily basis. Three and four episodes a day are not unusual, with 30 to 40 hot flashes a day occurring in severe cases. Other women may have several hot flashes during the night. When hot flashes recur throughout the night, sleep is often disturbed. Many women wake up from a sound sleep feeling hot and perspiring profusely. Often it is difficult to go back to sleep. Women with menopause-related insomnia may feel exhausted during the day because of sleep deprivation. Insomnia is a very common reason for women to visit their doctors seeking relief.

Other Vasomotor Symptoms

Women who have hot flashes often have other symptoms as well. Like hot flashes, these symptoms are due to vasomotor instability (varying degrees of vasoconstriction and vasodilatation of the blood vessels) and thus are considered to arise from the same cause. Such symptoms may present odd sensations that can be quite worrisome to women who do not understand that they are menopause related; for most women, they diminish in time. These symptoms include nausea, dizziness, faintness and palpitations (rapid and forceful heartbeats). Some women notice strange sensations of numbness and tingling in their arms and fingers. An unusual symptom is formication which women describe as a crawling feeling all over their skin. Luckily, this is not a common symptom.

Luckily, hot flashes do not last forever for most women. For half of the menopausal women who experience these symptoms, hot flash symptoms disappear within a year. For another 30 percent of women, they last up to two and one-half years. Unfortunately, however, for 20 percent of women, the hot flashes and other vasomotor symptoms can last five to ten years or even longer.

Cause of Hot Flashes

The cause of hot flashes is unclear, but it may be related to the decrease in estrogen output at the time of menopause. The pituitary gland responds to the drop in estrogen and progesterone by increasing its level of gonadotrophins, FSH and LH, in an effort to elevate estrogen and progesterone levels. The pituitary, in turn, is stimulated by releasing factors from the hypothalamus, which also regulates temperature control. As a result, the hormonal instability occurring at this time may also cause the "thermostat" in the brain to be reset downward with menopause. Another hypothesis is that hot flashes occur when the estrogen receptors in the hypothalamus do not receive enough estrogenic stimulation. In response, they may release a chemical substance that produces the hot flashes and other vasomotor responses.

Whatever the mechanism, lack of estrogen appears to play a major part in producing hot flashes, through its role in nervous system function and its effect on blood vessels. Research studies show that estrogen both excites and inhibits warm and cold sensitive nerve cells in the hypothalamus. Estrogen and progesterone are known to affect body temperature during the menstrual cycle. In blood vessels, estrogen can moderate vascular tone and affect how blood flow is distributed to various parts of the body. Women with hot flashes have higher blood flow to their forearm than women without hot flashes. Once they are treated with estrogen, the forearm blood flow diminishes. This may explain why treatment with HRT is so effective in reducing hot flash symptoms.

Hot Flash Triggers

Although the main cause of hot flashes appears to be the hormonal and nervous system instability that occurs at the time of menopause, other factors such as environment, emotions and diet can also trigger hot flashes. Women often report that the intensity and frequency of hot flashes increase in warm weather. During the worst heat of the summer, women may stand in front of air conditioners or open refrigerator doors to find relief. Often they wear as few layers of clothing as possible. Many women keep a thermos of ice-cold water or other beverage close by to cool themselves down.

Stress often brings on hot flashes. Patients report that the incidence of hot flashes increases dramatically before a talk or formal presentation, before a trip, during times of job or family stress, or even with strenuous exercise. In addition, the use of alcohol or caffeinated foods and beverages such as coffee, black tea, cola drinks and chocolate can trigger hot flashes because they tend to dilate the small blood vessels. Spicy food or hot drinks may have the same effect. Women who suffer from frequent and intense hot flashes should endeavor to keep a calm and peaceful mindset and practice meditation or relaxation techniques. They should also pay close attention to their diet during this period. Many self-help techniques to relieve hot flashes are discussed in Part II of this book.

HRT for Hot Flashes

Many studies using estrogen, progestins and estro-gen-progestin combinations show hormonal therapy effective in treating hot flashes and vasomotor symptoms. This is certainly validated in clinical practice because HRT is the most commonly prescribed treatment for hot flashes in the United States today.

Estrogen oral tablets in doses of 0.625 mg or an estro-gen transdermal patch in doses 0.05 mg is commonly used. Physicians consider this a moderate dose. Some women need a significantly higher dose for symptom relief. (Unfortunately, the higher doses can also cause more side effects.) Occasionally, even a low dosage of Premarin (0.3 mg) relieves hot flashes in women with mild symptoms.

Women who have had surgical menopause and no longer have a uterus can use estrogen alone. Women with an intact uterus may choose to take a progestin. It is normally taken with estrogen on a continuous basis, using low doses such as 2.5 mg per day. Alternatively, the progestin can be taken for 10 to 12 days per month in doses varying between 5 to 10 mg per day.

Progestin alone may be used by women who cannot use estrogen or do not tolerate it well because of side effects. Although the use of progestins alone is not as effective in suppressing hot flashes as combined estrogen-progestin therapy, it still helps many women. Most women take progestins as oral tablets, but in one research study an injectable form of progestin called Depo-Provera was found to relieve hot flashes in 89.5 percent of the women. Side effects, however, were fairly significant and included abnormal bleeding, headaches, vaginal dryness and depression.

Other Medical Therapies for Hot Flashes

One early form of treatment for hot flashes was phenobarbital, a strong sleep-inducing medication. This was researched primarily in the 1960s. Studies showed that 66 to 82 percent of the women subjects felt the drug provided symptom relief. Unfortunately, side effects and even habituation are problems with phenobarbital, and it was replaced in common use by HRT.

In more recent years, clonidine, a drug used to treat high blood pressure has been used for women who are not good candidates for HRT, including those who cannot use progesterone alone. Clonidine, however, is not nearly as effective in reducing hot flashes as HRT or ERT. One study found it to be effective in only 46 percent of the women who used it. In addition, some women discontinued the use of clonidine because of side effects such as nausea, fatigue and irritability. However, it may be worth a try if your hot flashes are severe and you wish to pursue medical therapy or if alternative therapies have not been successful.

Some physicians may prescribe tranquilizers such as Valium (which suppress hypothalamic function) or sedatives (which decrease autonomic nervous system irritability) to reduce vasomotor symptoms and insomnia. However, tranquilizers and sedatives can cause side effects including drowsiness and decreased mental acuity during the day and can be addicting with long-term use. As a result, these drugs should be used cautiously and only on a short-term basis.

Vaginal &
Bladder Aging

The reduced estrogen and androgen output by the ovaries after menopause causes the vagina and bladder to age dramatically, compromising their ability to function normally. Unlike hot flashes, mood swings and other early symptoms of menopause that tend to diminish over time, the symptoms of vaginal and bladder aging increase. As the years pass, they can cause women severe discomfort.

After a discussion of these changes and the symptoms that can result, information will be presented about the many helpful therapies that relieve these symptoms. Some therapies even reverse the signs of tissue aging and return the vagina and bladder to more youthful and healthful states.

Vaginal and Bladder Changes
After Menopause

With the onset of menopause, estrogen levels can drop by as much as 75 percent. As mentioned earlier, estrogen causes dilation and relaxation of the blood vessels, promoting good blood circulation to the organs and tissues throughout the body. When estrogen levels dwindle, blood flow to the genitals decreases. The tissues lose their pink or rosy color and, over time, become more pale. The vagina has many estrogen receptors, so its tissues are very responsive to the levels of hormones available. When estrogen is deficient, the vaginal and urethral linings lose their thick protective layer of surface cells and become thinner, drier and less elastic. They are much more easily injured and traumatized.

One of the earliest signs of vaginal aging is loss of lubrication. The cervix and vagina secrete much less mucus. How soon this occurs depends on how much estrogen the body makes after menopause. Within five years of menopause, 25 percent of women suffer from vaginal dryness because their ovaries and adrenals lose the ability to make sufficient estrogen to support these tissues. In other women whose bodies continue to make small but helpful amounts of estrogen, it may take as long as ten years before vaginal dryness becomes a problem. But eventually, it occurs in all women. An active sex life does help to maintain vaginal health and keep dryness to a minimum for a longer time.

Although vaginal and urethral dryness and a tendency toward being easily traumatized and irritated are early signs of vaginal and bladder aging, these are by no means the only indications. With time, the vagina actually shrinks and becomes shorter and narrower at the opening. The vaginal walls become less elastic. Patients have told me that they approach sex cautiously because their vaginal opening is so narrowed that penetration is quite painful.

Symptoms of Vaginal and Bladder Aging

As you can imagine, these changes in the vagina and bladder cause uncomfortable symptoms that affect normal function. These symptoms include vaginal soreness and painful intercourse, loss of sexual desire, vaginal and bladder infections and stress incontinence.

Vaginal Soreness
and Painful Intercourse

With the thinning and narrowing of the vagina, penetration by an object can be a painful experience. Many women find that their annual pelvic examination and PAP smear become quite an uncomfortable ordeal; the introduction of a vaginal speculum can be painful. The doctor may need to use a small, narrow speculum usually used for examining young girls. Insertion of fingers, a penis or other objects during sexual activity can be equally uncomfortable. The vagina can become easily irritated and sore with any form of penetration. The thrusting of the penis inside an atrophied vagina can cause excessive friction and discomfort. Many women experience a mild burning sensation, or in more severe cases, even a tearing sensation during intercourse. A few patients have told me they felt their vaginal walls were being ripped apart. Some women may experience increased bladder irritability with intercourse and may need to urinate.

Loss of Sexual Desire

In many women, vaginal pain and discomfort due to atrophic changes can cause a loss of sexual desire. Until the problem is treated and solved, these women, not surprisingly, try to avoid sex. Even women who formerly enjoyed sex may make excuses or stay away from intimate situations in which they may feel compelled to engage in sexual activity. If the husband or male partner wishes to maintain frequent episodes of lovemaking, lack of interest on the woman's part can create a great deal of stress in the relationship. (In other circumstances, I have seen stress occur when the woman is interested in sex and her male partner isn't. Relationships tend to suffer when the sexual interests of both parties differ greatly.)

In addition to the physical changes that make sexual activity uncomfortable, lack of hormonal support also decreases sexual arousal and sexual desire. Many postmenopausal women report a decrease in frequency and intensity of orgasm. Clitoral sensitivity can decline, as does the sensitivity of the cervix to a deep thrusting of the penis. Women may find their enjoyment of sex greatly diminished after menopause. As a result, frequency of sexual intercourse may decrease to less than once a month. Many of these physical changes are due to decreased estrogen stimulation of the nerve cells and blood vessels. Both nerve cells and blood vessels contain high levels of estrogen receptors. Lack of estrogen causes poor circulation to the genital region and decreased nerve response during sexual intercourse (or any sexual activity).

The availability of testosterone has a very strong effect on sexual desire or libido. Testosterone is produced during our active reproductive years by both the ovaries and the adrenals. Ten to 20 percent of women experience a drop in libido soon after ceasing menstruation; this is because their ovaries stop making testosterone as well as estrogen. In other women, the drop in testosterone may not occur until some years after menopause. As a result, their sexual desire may not decrease as rapidly and their libido may stay intact for some years. In fact, some women (approximately 10 percent) report an increase in libido after menopause. Some women find the lack of fear about becoming pregnant and the absence of menstruation quite liberating; they enjoy the increased sexual freedom without having to worry about birth control. Some women (and men) find that the increased privacy that occurs when children leave home (which can occur prior to or around the time of menopause) brings more sexual enjoyment, frequency and spontaneity in a home now shared primarily by the couple.

Vaginal and Bladder Infections

Vaginal infections can occur frequently in postmenopausal women because of the thinning and drying of the vaginal lining. The lining becomes easily irritated and injured, and as a result, it becomes very susceptible to infections by unhealthy organisms such as yeast and bacteria. The lack of estrogen support also causes the vaginal pH to change from acidic to alkaline. Healthy organisms such as lactobacillus thrive in an acidic environment, while the growth of harmful fungi and bacteria is inhibited. When the pH becomes too alkaline, the reverse occurs. Our normal healthy bacteria die off and are replaced by organisms that thrive in an alkaline pH. These organisms infect the tissues and cause unpleasant symptoms such as vaginal discharge, burning and unpleasant odor. These infections may be difficult to eradicate and may recur frequently even after treatment. Many women develop symptoms every time they have sexual intercourse. This occurs because the trauma to the fragile tissues caused by penile penetration make the environment attractive to harmful pathological organisms.

Recurrent urinary tract infections can also be a difficult and unpleasant problem for many postmenopausal women. Standard medical textbooks state that 10 percent of these women suffer from recurrent infections and that the incidence of urine contaminated by unhealthy bacteria (without causing symptoms) is 25 percent. In fact, an estimated 10 to 15 percent of women over age 60 have frequent urinary tract infections. Why do so many urinary tract infections occur? First, with the loss of estrogen support, the urethra, a small tube near the vaginal opening through which urine leaves the body, becomes less flexible and elastic. Like the vagina, the walls of the urethra thin out and become drier with time. Because the urethra is located so near the vaginal opening, it can become easily irritated after sexual intercourse and is more prone to infection. However, urinary tract infections are common even in women who aren't sexually active. Other factors also play a role in this process. As women age, the lower urinary tract stops manufacturing anti-adherence factors which help prevent bacteria from attaching to the bladder wall. Common symptoms of urinary tract infection include urinary frequency, burning and itching. Women may have to urinate often but void only a small amount of urine. Occasionally, the infection travels from the urethra and bladder up to the kidneys and causes a severe infection that can require hospitalization.

Stress Incontinence

Estrogen helps maintain muscle tone and firmness. When the estrogen supply dwindles, the uterus, vagina and bladder can lose their tone; the ligaments that help support these organs also lose their tone. As a result, the bladder, rectum and uterus can drop or prolapse. If the bladder prolapses, it can bulge or pouch into the vagina; this condition is called a cystocele. When the bladder is involved, women may suffer from incontinence or an inability to control their flow of urine. They may leak urine when they laugh, cough or sneeze. Sometimes the loss of urine is enough to soil undergarments and women may need to wear a small pad. When the rectum bulges into the vagina, it is called a rectocele. Women with a rectocele may complain of constipation. When the uterus prolapses, women may have a sensation of fullness or heaviness in their pelvis because the uterus has dropped and is not suspended in its normal position.

Therapies for Relief of Vaginal and Bladder Aging

Several categories of treatment may result in the desired symptom relief for women suffering from atrophic changes. These include HRT, lubricants, physical activity including Kegel exercises, frequent sexual activity, and other supportive therapy.

Estrogen Replacement Therapy (ERT)

Estrogen therapy helps all symptoms of vaginal and bladder atrophy. In fact, estrogen is remarkable for the speed and effectiveness with which it can restore health to these systems. It is the most helpful treatment available for revitalizing vaginal and bladder tissue. When taken orally, transdermally or as a vaginal cream, it thickens the mucous membranes and other tissues, restores elasticity and even improves lubrication. It also helps return the pH of the vagina to a more healthful acidic environment. All these changes promote the growth of healthy organisms and discourage infection by pathogens. The incidence of both vaginal and urinary tract infections tends to drop dramatically once ERT is instituted, becoming similar to that of younger women who are prone to occasional episodes.

ERT is equally effective in restoring libido. By relieving the symptoms of pain and discomfort, it allows sexual activity to become enjoyable and comfortable again. ERT also helps restore clitoral and cervical sensation as well as orgasmic intensity and frequency. Both blood circulation to the genitals and nerve cell response to sex are improved. ERT also helps restore tone and elasticity to the pelvic muscles and may help reduce symptoms of incontinence (although women with severe symptoms, prolapse or incontinence may require surgery). Clearly, ERT provides many benefits for good vaginal and bladder health and normal functioning.

Many women with vaginal or bladder symptoms may choose just to use the vaginal cream locally, limiting their total body exposure to estrogen. The amount of estrogen absorbed into the blood stream is initially high, but declines rapidly as the tough, cornified (callouslike), vaginal cells begin to regenerate with estrogen use. This new outer layer of cells then provides a barrier to estrogen absorption so the total body exposure drops.

It is important to use the lowest dose of estrogen possible that relieves your symptoms. Many women use 1 mg twice weekly with excellent results. However, research in England and Denmark suggests that as small a dose as 0.125 to 0.25 mg per treatment will effectively reduce symptoms. Positive results of the therapy can often be seen very rapidly. Many women report significant changes within two weeks of beginning treatment. However, women with severe atrophy may need several months of therapy to realize the full benefit of the treatment.

If you use the vaginal cream only, be sure to take a course of progesterone therapy several times a year if your uterus is still intact. Estrogen vaginal cream used without progesterone can cause endometrial hyperplasia. The progesterone is important for cleaning out the uterine lining completely and preventing a buildup of cells. It is also important to have regular examinations by your physician if you use the cream, just as you would with any other from of ERT. If you have any unusual episodes of bleeding after starting estrogen vaginal cream, report this to your physician for careful investigation. Also, be sure not to use the cream just before sexual intercourse as a lubricant. This can cause your partner to absorb estrogen, which is certainly not a good idea. If you need more vaginal moisture with sexual activity, use a lubricant and apply the estrogen vaginal cream at a different time.

For women who have other symptoms of menopause in addition to the vaginal and bladder changes, the use of oral or transdermal estrogen is an even more powerful and effective way to take ERT. For women with severe symptoms, the oral or transdermal forms of estrogen can be combined with the vaginal cream until the symptoms diminish. The systemic form of ERT is particularly important for women concerned about their long-term risk of osteoporosis or heart attacks. The vaginal cream used alone will not provide this important type of protection.

If estrogen alone doesn't restore your libido, it can be combined with very low amounts of testosterone. My experience prescribing very low doses of testosterone to patients is that it rapidly restored their libido. Normally, one or two percent testosterone cream is applied topically to the genital tissues. Other physicians prescribe low-dose testosterone pills (less than 75 mg per month). With both scenarios, the incidence of side effects is low, although they can occur. Typical side effects of testosterone include facial hair growth, acne and weight gain. Of more serious concern is testosterone's adverse effects on blood lipids and liver function. If you choose testosterone therapy, have your physician monitor you closely so that any adverse effects will be recognized and dealt with rapidly.

Lubricants

The many excellent water-based lubricants currently on the market provide additional moisture for both partners when used vaginally or rubbed on the penis and can reduce the friction and discomfort of sexual intercourse if the tissues tend to be dry. Good products include Astroglide (Bio Film, Inc.)— a favorite with many of my patients—and K-Y Jelly (Johnson & Johnson), which can be squeezed from a tube or bottle. Some women prefer to use a newer product called Replens (Parke-Davis) which is a moisturizing gel inserted as a suppository; each application of Replens lasts for three days. It acts by plumping up the cells of the vaginal lining with moisture. In addition, Replens has an acidic pH which helps to protect against vaginal infections by discouraging the growth of unhealthy organisms.

Other women prefer to use massage oil or vitamin E liquid or suppositories for additional lubrication. Although both of these can be quite helpful, it is important to avoid vaginal use of other oil-based products, such as Vaseline or baby oil. Unlike vitamin E and massage oil which are vegetable-oil based, these petroleum-based products will coat the vaginal lining and inhibit the release of your own secretions. They can even put women at higher risk of vaginal infections. Products designed for vaginal lubrication are safer and more effective for regular use.

Pelvic Activity

As mentioned earlier, regular sexual activity promotes better blood circulation to the vagina, as well as better tone and elasticity of the pelvic muscles and increased lubrication. Sexual activity stimulates all aspects of pelvic health if engaged in at least once or twice a week. If you don't have a regular partner, consider masturbation. This provides a solution, as well as a good sexual outlet for many women. I have had patients who are sexually active with their husbands once or twice a week and also enjoy masturbation to satisfy their sexual needs. Some women find the use of mechanical aids such as vibrators helpful in achieving orgasm. If you wish more information about this topic, there are many excellent sex guides available that deal with this subject in excellent detail.

Local exercises of the pelvic area can improve bladder control and vaginal elasticity, even increasing sexual pleasure. Dr. Arnold Kegel developed a set of exercises in the 1940s that all women should practice during the menopausal years. The Kegel exercises strengthen the muscles that surround the urethra, vagina and anus. Women who do these exercises frequently find that they are more aware of their vagina, find sex more pleasurable and they report more sensation in the pelvic area. Women also notice less leaking of urine when they cough, sneeze or laugh.

The Kegel exercises are simple and easy to do; they can be done anywhere—sitting, standing or lying down. To practice these exercises:

- Draw up the vaginal muscles, hold for three seconds, then relax. Repeat ten times.

- Squeeze your vaginal muscles firmly, then alternately contract and relax the muscles as rapidly as you can. Repeat ten times.

Preventive Suggestions for Vaginal Infections

To prevent vaginal infections (vaginitis), you may find it helpful to use an acidophilus supplement to help colonize your intestinal tract and vagina with these helpful bacteria that thrive in an acid environment. Nondairy yogurt with live acidophilus cultures is available in most health food stores. This yogurt is made of soybeans, an excellent food for menopausal women (see the chapters on nutrition for menopausal women in the second part of this book). Don't binge on sugar, chocolate or alcohol, which can promote the overgrowth of candida and trigger vaginal yeast infections. Avoid local irritation by washing with nonperfumed soap and water. After a bowel movement, wipe from front to back to avoid contamination of the vaginal and urethral tissues by intestinal bacteria. Do not wear panty hose and clothes that are tight in the crotch area as these can irritate fragile tissues. Wear cotton undergarments instead of synthetic material, which does not allow for proper drainage or air circulation in the crotch area.

If an infection is developing or if you are prone to infections, douche gently with one to two tablespoons of white vinegar in a quart of warm water. Some women find that vitamin C helps prevent vaginal infections from developing.

Be aware when selecting your sexual partner that sexually transmitted diseases (STDs) are more prevalent than ever before, and more dangerous. A partner who has had sex with many other women is much more likely to be harboring an organism that can give you an infection. If you are concerned about this issue, or in fact, if you are in any relationship that has not been totally monogamous for the past several years, ask your partner to wear a condom.

Preventive Suggestions for Urinary Tract Infections

Good hygiene also helps prevent urinary tract infections. Be sure to wash daily using a nonperfumed or nonirritating soap and warm water and urinate several times a day. Holding your urine increases the chance of developing an infection. Drink plenty of water, at least eight glasses a day. Urinating more frequently prevents your urine from becoming very concentrated and helps flush out your bladder. Urinate immediately before and after sexual intercourse. Many women are more prone to both vaginal and urinary tract infections after sexual activity.

An acid environment is healthier for the urinary tract and tends to prevent infections more than an alkaline environment. Taking supplements of acidophilus, vitamin C and cranberry juice helps some women prevent infections. Cranberry juice contains compounds that prevent bacteria from sticking to the urinary tract wall. Do not drink cranberry juice that has been sweetened with added sugar; use only the tart, natural juice. One to two glasses per day should suffice. Don't drink more than this because the acidic juice may be irritating to the stomach lining. Soy yogurt with live acidophilus culture is a delicious and healthy food. Unfortunately, it is not available in most supermarkets, but can be found in many health food stores.

Some physicians prescribe a medication called Mandelamine which helps acidify urine and combat infections. Macrodantin and Septra antibiotics are other medications frequently prescribed by physicians to treat infections or as a long-term therapy to prevent infections. Currently, a topically applied intravaginal estriol cream has been useful in decreasing the incidence of infections. A study done in 1993 on 93 postmenopausal women concluded that the intravaginal administration of estriol prevented recurrent urinary tract infections, probably by modifying the vaginal flora. Often, however, estrogen therapy and the other preventive measures discussed in this chapter are the best ways to keep your urinary tract healthy and infection-free.

Symptoms of Vaginal and Bladder Aging

Vaginal soreness and painful intercourse
Loss of sexual desire
Vaginal and bladder infections
Stress incontinence

Therapies for Relief of Vaginal and Bladder Aging

Estrogen Replacement Therapy (ERT)
  Estrogen oral tablets, transdermal patch or vaginal cream
  Testosterone tablets or cream
Lubricants
Pelvic activity
  Sexual activity
  Kegel exercises
Preventive suggestions for vaginal infections
Preventive suggestions for urinary tract infections

7

Menopausal Mood Swings

*D*uring the menopause years, women may notice that their moods fluctuate more easily. Mood changes can vary from increased anxiety and irritability to depression and fatigue. Many women become distressed by these changes because they affect the quality of their personal relationships. Women report being bad tempered toward family, friends and co-workers and responding to daily life stresses in a more irritable fashion.

Many women describe these feelings as similar to the emotional ups and downs of premenstrual syndrome (PMS). A woman who has had PMS during her active reproductive years may be particularly distressed by her emotional fluctuations. Often, the expectation is that PMS symptoms will stop, rather than exacerbate, during the transition into menopause.

Luckily, not every woman experiences such pronounced emotional swings (in fact, some women go through menopause with no mood changes at all). However, if you are among those women who do, you will find very helpful information in this chapter on the causes of and treatments for menopausal mood swings.

Causes of Mood Swings are Complex

The complex causes of mood swings in most women can be due to hormonal changes, social and cultural factors, or more commonly, a combination of both. Some women are very sensitive to the rapid drop in their estrogen and progesterone levels that occurs with menopause. They may feel as if they are on an emotional roller-coaster as their hormones drop and readjust to a new, lower level. This is because estrogen and progesterone have a profound effect on the mood as well as the body. Progesterone has a sedative effect on the nervous system. When levels are too high, women may feel depressed and tired. On the other hand, estrogen has a stimulant effect on the nervous system, causing anxiety and irritability when estrogen output is elevated. Conversely, women may feel more depressed and moody when estrogen levels are diminished.

Under optimal conditions, estrogen output and progesterone output exist in a state of healthy equilibrium in the body. When you feel emotionally comfortable and you are not experiencing extreme mood fluctuations, these hormones are probably in balance. However, with the transition into menopause, hormonal levels shift rapidly, fluctuating between very high and low levels, then occasionally settling into balance again. Finally, both hormones drop permanently to low, postmenopausal levels. Likewise, moods may follow no obvious pattern, fluctuating as the hormones shift in sensitive women.

Unstable hormone levels can also affect how well we handle our daily life stresses. Research studies suggest that estrogen affects catecholamine levels in the body. Catecholamines are chemicals that affect the sympathetic nervous system. (This is the part of our nervous system that governs our "fight-or-flight" response or how our body deals with stress.) When the sympathetic nervous system is triggered, it causes muscles to tense, blood vessels to constrict, and heart and pulse rate to speed up to prepare for reacting to an emergency. Women in early menopause may find the fight-or-flight response more easily triggered in response to day-to-day stress. This may put them in a frequent state of tension. They tend to react to small stresses the same way they would react to emergencies. The energy that accumulates in the body to meet this "emergency" must then be discharged. Women may become upset and angry before, once again, the system comes into balance.

For women, the social and cultural factors occurring before, during and after menopause may be quite stressful and can contribute to their mood fluctuations. For some women, menopause may signal loss of reproduction which may be experienced as loss of usefulness. For other women, menopause is a time when children leave home and move away, major career changes are made or a marriage ends in divorce. The combination of hormonal and biochemical changes, plus lifestyle changes, can be quite difficult for many women to handle. Some women find themselves alone without their old familiar support systems intact during this time of transition. Other women find they have to cope with a husband's midlife crisis, engendered by loss of job or job dissatisfaction, health problems and other issues that are common for men around midlife. Some women become emotionally distressed at the bodily changes that menopause causes. Many women mention feeling unhappy with the wrinkles, loss of muscle tone and change in body shape that can occur very rapidly after menopause.

Solutions for Menopausal Mood Swings

Menopause-related mood swings can be relieved through a variety of therapeutic approaches. These include the use of HRT, mood-altering medications, counseling and support groups, and a variety of self-help methods. The first three of these methods are discussed in this chapter. More specific information on self-help methods is presented in Part II of this book.

Hormone Replacement Therapy

Research studies have shown that estrogen has a mood-elevating effect. Women on HRT may perceive this as a sense of well-being and overall mental balance that contributes to the relief of other menopausal symptoms such as hot flashes and vaginal dryness. My patients have been pleased when their emotions have been smoothed out; this occurs once they start hormonal therapy. The mood-elevating effects of estrogen are thought to be due to its effect on brain and nerve function.

Another benefit of estrogen is its positive effect on the quality of sleep. Estrogen improves REM (rapid eye movement) sleep. REM sleep is often disturbed in women who are hormonally deficient. Better sleep quality helps relieve the fatigue and depression from which some menopausal women suffer.

As previously discussed, estrogen improves short-term memory. Many menopausal women find that they forget things. Although usually of small significance in day-to-day functioning, this decrease in short-term memory can be quite distressing. Research studies show that the difference in short-term memory between postmenopausal women who use ERT versus those who do not is significant.

Estrogen is not the only hormone useful for mood fluctuations. Research studies have shown that testosterone has beneficial effects on emotional well-being, perhaps even more striking than those noted with ERT. In one controlled study of 43 women who had undergone surgical menopause with removal of both ovaries, women responded better to estrogen combined with testosterone than to ERT alone. Significant improvements were noted in emotional well-being, appetite and energy level. Testosterone used alone also had beneficial effects. However, when testosterone does not relieve hot flashes or other vasomotor symptoms, it is probably desirable to combine it with low doses of estrogen. Combined estrogen-testosterone therapy is not appropriate for all women. It is probably most useful in women who have undergone surgical removal of their ovaries (oophorectomy) or whose ovaries have stopped producing even small amounts of testosterone and estrogen soon after menopause.

Mood-Altering Drugs

Even though HRT can reduce the mood swings due to the hormonal changes at the time of menopause, it will not be an effective therapy for mood problems due to psychological disorders. Major depression or anxiety episodes may require medication developed specifically for these conditions. If your emotional symptoms are severe, request that your physician do a careful evaluation or send you for a psychological or psychiatric consultation to differentiate menopause-related emotional symptoms from those due to psychological conditions. This will enable the best and most effective therapies to be selected.

Two primary types of medications are used for psychologically-based mood disorders: benzodiazepine tranquilizers and sedatives, and antidepressants. The benzodiazepine tranquilizers include commonly prescribed drugs such as Xanax (alprazolam), Valium (diazepam), and Librium (chlordiazepoxide HCl). These drugs can be useful in relieving excessive anxiety, insomnia and irritability in menopausal women. The benzodiazepine sedatives include "sleeping pills" such as Dalmane (flurazepam), Halcion (triazolam), and Restoril (temazepam). These drugs, when used on a short-term basis, can help induce a state of deep sleep as well as reduce the number of hot flashes. However, they do not effectively relieve anxiety, irritability or mood swings. Benzodiazepine tranquilizers and sedatives must be used cautiously and only on a short-term basis. They may cause significant side effects such as drowsiness, a real problem if you need to drive or concentrate effectively. In addition, drug dependency can develop over time.

These drugs are not curative. Eighty percent of women report their anxiety symptoms return once the drugs are stopped. Although these drugs can relieve symptoms in the short-run, a combination of natural self-help therapies and counseling will help prevent a recurrence of anxiety symptoms on a long-term basis.

Antidepressants are used for menopausal women who have severe depression and fatigue symptoms. Other than Prozac, currently one of the most popular antidepressants with the least number of side effects, the antidepressant category of drugs used today is primarily tricyclics. These produce both antidepressant and mild tranquilizing effects. Building up to a therapeutic effect takes some time after initiation of treatment. After two to three weeks of treatment, however, 80 percent of depressed and anxious patients notice an elevation of mood, increased alertness, and improvement in appetite. Common tricyclic medications include Elavil (amitriptyline), Tofranil (imipramine), Sinequan (doxepin), Aventyl (nortriptyline), and Norpramin (desipramine). The actual mechanism of drug action is not known, but it is thought that depression is relieved by elevating the levels of neurotransmitters such as serotonin and norepinephrine. These are chemicals present in the brain that regulate mood, personality, sleep and appetite. Many women with depression lack adequate levels of these neurotransmitters.

As with tranquilizers and sedatives, side effects of these drugs are fairly common. As many as one-quarter of all patients stop such therapy because of these unpleasant side effects. Many women using antidepressants initially complain of dry mouth, blurred vision, constipation, drowsiness, or even anxiety and agitation. These symptoms tend to fade in intensity after the first few weeks. Sometimes initiating therapy at very low doses minimizes these symptoms. Another side effect is shakiness or tremors in the hands; this occurs in 10 percent of women. Numbness and tingling in the arms and legs are also occasionally reported.

Unlike the benzodiazepines, antidepressants are not physically addictive, so the threat of developing withdrawal symptoms is not an issue. Some women become psychologically addicted to the antidepressants, however, and may have a difficult time weaning themselves from the medication. As a result, it is best to use HRT, counseling, and self-help techniques as much as possible to treat emotional symptoms during the menopausal period. Although mood-altering medications can be very helpful, try to use them for the shortest period and in the lowest dosages that bring symptom relief.

Counseling Services and Support Groups

Many menopausal women gain tremendous relief from emotional distress by seeking psychological counseling, discussing issues with their health care providers or joining support groups. If you are not sure where to find these resources, call clinics and hospitals in your area offering women's programs. Often, they can refer you to national and local self-help groups that offer classes and other resources.

My perception is that women are seeking these resources in record numbers. There is currently an explosion in menopause-related workshops, seminars, classes and on-going support groups throughout the United States. Many of them offer additional social and emotional support to midlife women far beyond what most doctors' offices or clinics offer.

Medical Resources for Menopausal Mood Swings

Hormone Replacement Therapy
    Estrogen
    Testosterone
Mood-altering drugs
    Benzodiazepine tranquilizers
    Benzodiazepine sedatives
    Antidepressants
Counseling services and support groups

8

Osteoporosis & Other Physical Changes

One of the most serious consequences of post-menopausal aging is the development of osteoporosis. In fact, osteoporosis is a major health problem affecting more than 25 million older Americans, 90 percent of them women. One out of three American women will develop osteoporosis, probably after menopause.

The statistics surrounding osteoporosis are astounding. More than 1.3 million fractures occur each year as a result of this condition. Eighty percent of the 250,000 hip fractures in the United States each year occur in women over age 65 as a result of osteoporosis. About one-quarter of these women die within one year from complications, such as blood clots and pneumonia, caused by their convalescence. Another one-third never regain the ability to function physically or socially on their own. These women spend the rest of their lives requiring long-term care in nursing facilities. In addition to causing hip fractures, osteoporosis is also responsible for loss of bone in the jaw, gum recession (both of which are early signs of this condition), dowager's hump, loss of height, back pain due to compression and fractures of the vertebra, and fractures of the wrist (called colles fractures by physicians).

Often these fractures occur when only mild stress is put on the bone. This can include missing a step and falling down, falling on an extended arm or lifting a heavy object. Because of the underlying weakness of the bone, fractures can also occur spontaneously without any preceding trauma. This often occurs with vertebral fractures.

This chapter will discuss what happens to bones with osteoporosis, risk factors for osteoporosis, diagnosis of osteoporosis and other structural changes associated with menopause. Finally, therapies for osteoporosis and other structural changes will be explored.

What Happens to Bones with Osteoporosis

Bones are living tissue; we are constantly forming new bone cells to add to our skeletal mass and removing old cells that are no longer useful. This simultaneous addition and subtraction of bone from our skeleton is called bone remodeling; from five to ten percent of our bone is replaced through this process every year. Bone remodeling involves two types of bone cells. Osteoblasts create new bone cells, while osteoclasts are responsible for removing old cells from the skeleton. This delicately balanced process is carefully regulated by many of the hormones in our body such as estrogen, progesterone, calcitonin and thyroid (as well as other hormones).

During the first 30 to 35 years of life, we deposit more bone in our skeleton than we lose, provided our health status is normal. In fact, our bone mass is at its peak in our 20s and begins to decrease in the mid-30s. According to peak bone mass theory, our bones reach their peak level of healthy density by the early 20s. The more healthy our bones are at this stage, the less risk of osteoporosis later in life. In the years preceding menopause, bone loss begins to exceed the addition of new bone to the skeleton. As a result, bones begin to lose important minerals such as calcium as well as their matrix or intracellular substance. This causes a decrease in bone density as well as an increased brittleness or porousness of the bones.

Initially, this process occurs very slowly, and women are not even aware that it is going on. However, with loss of hormonal support to the bones at the time of menopause, this process accelerates. The first years after the onset of menopause can be a time of rapid bone loss for many women unless they have instituted therapies that emphasize prevention. Bone is lost at the rate of one to three percent per year for five to ten years after menopause. If the process of bone loss continues unabated, osteoporosis may eventually result. Unfortunately, most women are unaware that they are losing bone during their early postmenopausal years. By the time osteoporosis becomes apparent as they begin to suffer from pain and fractures, women are already in their 60s or 70s. Older women with osteoporosis may have lost as much as 40 to 45 percent of their total bone mass.

Men also start to lose bone mass around age 40 (approximately three to five percent per decade). However, they have thicker bones to start with; men have approximately 30 percent more bone mass than women. In addition, the male hormone, testosterone, helps maintain bone mass and strength. Both estrogen in women and testosterone in men help control calcium absorption by the bones. These hormones prevent the resorption of calcium from the bones into the blood circulation where calcium can be excreted from the body. However, unlike women whose estrogen levels drop precipitously at menopause, men can maintain their testosterone levels well into old age. As a result, their bones remain thicker and stronger many more years than those of women. This translates into more osteoporosis-related fractures for women than men—eight times more hip fractures and ten times more wrist fractures.

Although gender and age contribute greatly to the fractures that occur in old age because of osteoporosis, these are not the only factors. Many physicians also attribute fractures in the elderly to poor balance and lack of ability to right oneself when tripping or stumbling. Many older people lack flexibility, so when they fall, they absorb a much greater shock than if they could cushion themselves effectively or right themselves quickly. As a result, hip fractures increase with age, mirroring the loss of agility that occurs for many elderly women (and men).

Risk Factors for Osteoporosis

Not all women have the same risk of developing osteoporosis. Some women maintain strong and heavy bones throughout their lives, while other women develop accelerated bone loss soon after menopause. If you suspect you are at risk of developing osteoporosis, become knowledgeable about which factors have been linked to a higher incidence of this disease. This will help you and your physician evaluate your risk when planning an optimal treatment program. These factors include racial background, family history, hormonal status, lifestyle habits and pre-existing health conditions.

Racial Background

Skin pigmentation appears to parallel bone mass. African-American women are less likely to develop osteoporosis than white women. In fact, women at the highest risk are small and fair-skinned. These are typically women of Northern European ancestry such as Dutch, German or English background with blond, reddish or light brown hair and pale skin. Oriental women have a higher risk of developing osteoporosis, too. Even among similar groups, the risk is lower with women who have darker skin. For example, in Israel the darker skin Sephardic Jews have a lower rate of fractures than do Jewish women of European origin.

Family History

If your close female relatives suffered from osteoporosis, you have a higher risk of developing this problem. Many women have seen their mothers or grandmothers develop a dowager's hump or become disabled after suffering a hip fracture. This can be quite upsetting for the entire family who must deal with the long-term disability.

Hormonal Status

The age at which women begin menopause and how much hormonal support they maintain during their postmenopausal years affects bone density. Women who have had a surgical menopause before age 40 with removal of their ovaries are at high risk of osteoporosis because of the abrupt withdrawal of estrogen at a young age. Similarly, women who go through an early natural menopause are at high risk. A woman going through early menopause at age 35 or 40 has as much as 10 to 15 years less estrogen protection for her bones than a woman going through menopause at age 50. Thus, the older you are when going through menopause, the more years of hormonal protection are provided for your bones.

Although obesity is a health risk for many diseases such as osteoarthritis and uterine cancer, being overweight does offer some protection against osteoporosis in postmenopausal women. This is because the fat cells produce a type of estrogen called estrone through conversion of an adrenal hormone called androstenedione. This type of estrogen provides some support for the bones once the ovarian source of estrogen has dwindled.

Lifestyle Habits

Women who engage in regular physical exercise and are more muscular have a lower risk of developing osteoporosis. Physical activity also helps keep women flexible and agile which reduces the likelihood of fractures. Conversely, inactivity increases your risk. Young women and men confined to bed for long periods show a decrease in bone mass.

Many nutritional factors affect your risk of developing osteoporosis, too. Women who drink more than two cups of coffee per day or large amounts of other caffeine-containing beverages such as black tea or colas, or who consume more than two alcoholic drinks per day, are at higher risk. Smokers also run a higher risk of osteoporosis. High protein or salt intake are risk factors, as is inadequate calcium intake. When you do not have an adequate intake of calcium, the body takes it from your bones to maintain a blood level necessary for various processes such as heart rhythm and blood clotting.

Pre-Existing Health Issues

Women with a history of bulimia, anorexia or malabsorption syndrome have an increased risk of poor calcium absorption or low estrogen levels (often the case in women with anorexia who do not have a body fat level high enough to produce adequate estrogen). Women who use thyroid medication, suffer from an overactive thyroid gland, or use cortisone for a variety of chronic conditions are at higher risk. This is also true of women with chronic kidney disease. All these conditions can adversely affect calcium balance in the body.

Risk Factors for Osteoporosis

Membership in a nonblack ethnic group

Fair, pale skin color

Having female relatives with osteoporosis

Early menopause (before age 40)

Being short and thin

Childlessness

High alcohol use (more than 5 ounces per day)

High caffeine use

Smoking

Low calcium diet

Lack of vitamin D

High-salt diet

High-protein diet

Chronic diarrhea or surgical removal of stomach or
small intestine

Lactose deficiency

Daily use of cortisone

Use of thyroid medication (over 2 grains), Dilantin, or
aluminum-containing antacids

Uremia (kidney disease)

Diagnosis of Osteoporosis

If you are not sure about the status of your bones, excellent tests are available to evaluate the likelihood of developing osteoporosis. A new, low-dose x-ray test allows physicians to diagnose osteoporosis in the early stages before the bone loss is so severe that fractures occur. DEXA bone densitometry is a safe and painless procedure that assesses bone mineral density of the lumbar spine and hip, using 1/10 the x-ray of a single chest film. Another test is the computerized axial tomography (also called a CAT scan), which can measure bone density in the spine. The CAT scan uses higher x-ray dosages and is a more expensive test. These tests are much more sensitive than conventional x-ray, which can detect osteoporosis only when 25–40 percent or more of the bone mass is lost.

You may choose to have a bone density test done if you are trying to decide whether or not to use HRT. If the tests show accelerated bone loss for your age group, you should seriously consider the use of HRT unless other major health issues contraindicate the use of hormones.

Another test for osteoporosis is the Pyridinoline Cross Links assay, a simple urine test that measures cross-linking amino acids, the breakdown of collagen products. These are excreted in the urine in increased amounts and act as biochemical markers of systemic bone loss with osteoporosis.

Other Structural Changes Associated With Menopause

The loss of hormonal support affects not only the bones and teeth but other structural elements of the body such as the joints, muscles, body shape, skin and hair. Although bone loss may occur silently for many years, women notice changes in these other structural elements within a few years of entering menopause.

For instance, the incidence of osteoarthritis increases at the time of menopause; women who have never experienced joint pain suddenly become symptomatic. In addition, women with pre-existing arthritis find that their symptoms get worse. Many women reaching menopause complain of increased stiffness in their hands and shoulders as well as low back pain.

The lack of sex hormones also affects muscle tone. Muscles throughout the body tend to sag and lose tone after menopause. Women tend to be very conscious of pelvic muscle tone loss, as well as sagging of the facial and arm muscles. The loss of pelvic muscle tone can affect sexual pleasure and the ability to hold urine. Facial drooping can appear fairly rapidly within a year or two of menopause. This change can be a cause of distress in many women who don't like this visible sign of aging. Other tissues, such as the breasts, lose their tone and droop more. The lack of estrogen is probably also responsible for the increase in low back and pelvic pain that women experience around this time.

Another visible sign of aging for many women after menopause is a change in body shape as the distribution of weight on the body changes. The waist and upper back get thicker, while the hips and breasts tend to lose some of their fat. The result is that the female shape changes from an hourglass figure to a pear shape. Many women find that not only does their figure shape change, but they gain weight more easily (10 to 15 pounds in the year or two following menopause isn't unusual). This can occur no matter how diligently they diet or how much they exercise. The lack of female hormonal support plus the slowing of the metabolism are probably responsible for these changes. Women after menopause don't burn calories as efficiently as during their younger years. Careful attention to diet and regular exercise can certainly help, if not entirely correct, these physical changes. Examine the self-help chapters in this book for more in-depth information.

The skin and hair undergo many changes after menopause due to loss of estrogen. There is a gradual tendency toward thinning and dryness of the skin. Skin pigmentation becomes uneven which affects coloration. Some women may lose their even skin tone and notice patches of lighter and darker skin. As collagen production in the skin slows down, the skin loses its elasticity. The underlying muscle and fat tissues that help give skin its underlying support begin to shrink. There is also a reduction in sweat gland activity and decreased tolerance to temperature changes. As a result, many visible signs of skin aging become apparent such as pronounced wrinkling and creasing. Many women find these changes cosmetically unappealing and employ a variety of dermatologic aids in an attempt to make their skin look younger and healthier.

Women who smoke, have poor nutritional habits or have had excessive exposure to sunlight are more likely to show signs of skin aging at a younger age. Conversely, women who tend to carry a little extra weight or have reached menopause at a later age will have better looking skin. This is because they have had higher circulating levels of estrogen in their bodies for more years than a thin woman who enters menopause at an early age.

Lack of estrogen also affects the hair. With menopause, hair on the head and in the pubic area becomes drier, coarser and sparser. Women may also notice the growth of darker or coarser hair in areas where they've never had hair before, such as the chin, upper lip, chest or abdomen. This unusual growth of hair is due to the stimulation of the hair follicle by low amounts of androgens, a type of male hormone. High estrogen levels block the action of these male hormones on hair follicle receptors. However, after menopause, these low amounts of androgen may not decrease to the same extent that estrogen does in certain women. These unopposed androgens can then affect the pattern of hair growth and hair loss, taking on a more malelike pattern.

Therapies for Osteoporosis and Other Structural Changes

Osteoporosis and other age-related changes in the joints, muscles, skin and hair can be treated through the use of HRT. Other medications and supportive measures may also play a useful supporting role for certain conditions.

Hormone Replacement Therapy

Medical studies show that hormonal therapy not only helps prevent osteoporosis but also protects women against further bone loss. Both estrogen and progestins by themselves are protective, but used together they may provide benefits exceeding the use of either hormone alone. A Danish study done in 1991 showed that a combination of estrogen and a progestogen given no later than three years after the onset of menopause completely prevented bone loss in 18 women. In contrast, untreated women suffered significant bone loss.

Hormonal replacement therapy with conjugated estrogens (Premarin) at a dose of 0.625 mg per day has been shown to prevent osteoporosis in 90 percent of postmenopausal women who had no pre-existing osteoporosis. However, in one study done by Dr. Bruce Ettenger, even minimal estrogen supplementation (0.3 mg) prevented bone loss. If osteoporosis is already present, then a high dosage of estrogen is utilized, normally 1.25 to 2.5 mg per day. The estrogen oral tablet and transdermal patch appear to be equally effective in preventing bone loss. The vaginal cream should not be used for this purpose because absorption into the bloodstream may be erratic.

Various studies comparing women using estrogen with control women not on ERT showed significant differences in bone health. In one study done in Scotland by Dr. Robert Lindsay, women on ERT maintained their normal stature, while control women had a significant loss of height. Another study of 1,000 women treated with ERT for 15 years found a 70 percent reduction in wrist fractures from the expected rate. Even more striking was the observation that no hip fractures were seen in these women over the same 15-year period. A study was done at the Mayo Clinic comparing vertebral fracture rate in postmenopausal women treated with various combinations of estrogen, calcium and sodium fluoride. The group utilizing ERT had by far the lowest rate of vertebral fractures.

Estrogen appears to protect the bones through several mechanisms. Estrogen reduces urinary calcium and hydroxy-proline excretion which suggests it inhibits osteoclast function, the cells that break down bone tissue. Current research suggests that estrogen may even have a stimulatory effect on osteoblast cells, the cells that build up new bone. Estrogen also facilitates calcium absorption from the intestinal tract and increases parathyroid hormone and calcitonin production. The parathyroid hormone facilitates calcium absorption, while calcitonin stimulates bone formation. Estrogen appears to be critical to bone remodeling; therefore, it may well be the most essential component of prevention for osteoporosis.

The question of how long to stay on ERT is an important one for many women. Although the research data on this issue is not yet definitive, women who want to protect their bones from developing osteoporosis should consider using ERT at least ten years, possibly for life. Ideally, estrogen should be started within three years of the last menstrual period. Women already showing accelerated bone loss and considered at high risk for osteoporosis should probably make a lifetime commitment to ERT.

The longer you use ERT, the more protection your bones will have. As soon as you stop using it, your bones will begin to show signs of calcium loss and bone aging. It is never too late to begin estrogen therapy. Women in their 80s and 90s who had pre-existing osteoporosis showed some benefit after starting estrogen therapy. According to one recent study, supplemental hormones benefited women 15 years after initial diagnosis of osteoporosis. In another study, estrogen therapy increased vertebral bone mass and bone density at the femoral head. Interestingly, the best response was in women farthest away from menopause who had the lowest bone mass. ,

The addition of a progestin to the estrogen therapy may provide even better benefits. Though estrogen alone helps protect against calcium loss, at least eight medical studies suggest that the use of estrogen and a progestin in combination has the additional benefit of increasing bone mass by promoting new bone formulation. Recent research has led to the conclusion that progesterone acts directly to stimulate new bone by attaching to the osteoblast cell receptors. Progesterone also appears to increase bone turnover. Animal studies found that bone volume was greater in animals receiving both hormones than those who received only estrogen.

One study followed women using cyclic estrogen-progestin and women receiving a placebo for a ten-year period. Women who began the combined therapy within three years of entering menopause showed an increase in bone density throughout the entire study period. Women who began HRT later than three years following the onset of menopause showed some demineralization but much less than the placebo group. This study underlines the importance of beginning HRT in the early stages of menopause.

Another study compared the effects of estrogen therapy alone with combined estrogen-progestin therapy on the metabolic parameters of bone. This included measurements of the blood level and the urinary calcium/creatinine ratio. All values decreased (indicating decreased calcium excretion) with the use of estrogen. The addition of a progestin, however, decreased these values even more, showing substantial bone protection.

In addition to protecting bone, HRT has been shown to help reduce symptoms of osteoarthritis. As mentioned earlier, joint pain tends to become worse in early menopause. Many women with muscle and joint pain, including low back and pelvic pain, note relief of these symptoms within two weeks of beginning HRT. As an additional side benefit, HRT may provide protection against developing rheumatoid arthritis. Reported in the *Journal of the American Medical Association*, one study found that there was a greater than three-fold reduced incidence of rheumatoid arthritis in 1,000 women who had taken HRT compared with those who had not taken HRT.

HRT may also benefit postmenopausal women suffering from loss of muscle tone and firmness. If these effects are particularly pronounced in the pelvic area, urinary incontinence or uterine, bladder or urethral prolapse may result. HRT helps restore muscle tone and may relieve mild symptoms of incontinence and prolapse. However, women with severe cases may still require more drastic therapy, such as surgery. As mentioned earlier, muscle pain may accompany joint pain, particularly in the low back. HRT may help relieve more generalized muscle aches and pains, too.

Although estrogen will not restore skin to its youthful appearance, it can have a significant impact on skin quality. Women on estrogen therapy usually have thicker, oilier, moister and firmer skin. ERT improves subcutaneous fat deposition, which makes the skin tighter, and collagen turnover, which thickens and firms up the skin. Estrogen also increases fluid retention in the skin, making it look moister and plumper. However, to improve skin condition estrogen should be started soon after entering menopause because it cannot completely reverse any significant skin damage that has already occurred.

ERT does not have quite as dramatic an effect on the hair, but it will balance the androgen levels in the body again. As a result, unwanted hair on chin, chest and abdomen will stop growing. Once a woman has started ERT, these hairs can be pulled out and will not regrow as long as estrogen therapy continues.

Other Therapies for Healthy Bones

Other drugs have been used besides HRT to prevent bone loss and protect against the development of osteoporosis. Some therapies have been found more effective than others.

Sodium Fluoride

Fluoride has been studied as a preventive therapy for osteoporosis with mixed results. On the positive side, people living in areas in which the water has a high-fluoride content have higher average bone density than people living in a low-fluoride area. However, according to studies done using supplemental fluoride therapy in postmenopausal women, different types of bone show unequal changes in response to fluoride. A study done by the Mayo Clinic found that fluoride therapy increases bone density in one type of bone, called trabecular bone, but decreases cortical bone density. This may increase skeletal fragility and increase the risk of hip fractures. As a result of this study, the Mayo Clinic abandoned the use of fluoride therapy. Fluoride therapy may also cause other side effects such as anemia and intestinal disturbances.

Etidronate Disodium (Didronel)

Didronel has been used to treat women with osteoporosis who are at high risk of developing vertebral fractures and deformity. This drug coats the bone cells and specifically helps to prevent further bone loss in the spine. It has even been found to reverse some of the spinal damage that osteoporosis causes. Etidronate does not appear, however, to reverse damage in the hips, femur and other bones. In addition, some studies indicate that women who took this drug experience a higher rate of fractures than those who did not. However, this drug is continuing to be studied. Etidronate is usually administered daily for two weeks, followed by daily calcium supplementation for ten to twelve weeks. The treatment regimen is repeated every three months.

Other Supportive Measures

Besides the use of HRT and drugs, there are many actions a woman can take to prevent damage to her bones, joints, muscles, skin and hair after menopause. Healthy lifestyle habits can slow down the aging of all these bones and tissues, helping them remain healthy and at peak function. These beneficial measures include the following.

- Do regular weight-bearing exercise such as walking or weight training at least thirty minutes per day. This helps keep bones strong and intact and promotes good blood circulation.

- Practice yoga or other stretching exercises to keep your joints and muscles limber and flexible.

- Limit cigarette use and alcohol intake.

- Avoid sun exposure unless you use a high SPF sunscreen (15 or more). The sun causes damage and aging of the skin if protection from its rays is not used regularly.

- Drink lots of water—at least eight glasses per day—to thoroughly hydrate your skin and other tissues.

- Apply moisturizers to your skin to help lock in the fluid.

- Lose weight slowly if you diet. Rapid weight loss can accelerate the aging of your skin's appearance.

- Avoid overprocessing your hair with permanents and other hair care techniques that can cause excessive dryness and splitting of the hair.

- If you want to have unwanted hair removed, consider electrolysis. This is the only permanent method for hair removal. It is important, however, to work with an experienced and knowledgeable operator. Your health care practitioner can probably recommend an operator in your community.

Structural Components of the Body
That Show Menopausal Changes

Bones

Joints

Muscles

Skin

Hair

Treatment Options for Osteoporosis

Hormone replacement therapy
   Estrogen
   Progestins
   Estrogen-progestin combinations
Drugs
   Sodium fluoride
   Etidronate Disodium (Didronel)
General supportive measures

9

Estrogen Therapy & Risk of Heart Disease and Stroke

Coronary heart disease is the main killer of American women, claiming the lives of more than a quarter of a million women per year. More women die from heart disease than die from all forms of cancer. Although younger women also die of heart disease, it occurs less frequently during the active reproductive years. The incidence of heart disease escalates as women age. From age 30 to 60, cancer is the main cause of death in women, with heart disease in second place from age 40 to 60. Over age 60, heart disease becomes the leading cause of death in women.

Most women die from heart attacks due to coronary artery disease, where there is a narrowing of one or more of the arteries that supplies blood and oxygen to the heart. This narrowing is caused by the formation of plaque in the arteries. Plaque is a thick, waxy, yellowish substance consisting primarily of cholesterol, smooth muscle cells and foam cells. As the formation of plaque progresses, it can obstruct the flow of blood through the blood vessels. Over time, this will seriously compromise function of the heart, finally leading to a heart attack. Unfortunately, the obstruction is usually quite advanced before it begins to cause symptoms of chest pain, angina and shortness of breath on mild exertion.

General Risk Factors for Heart Disease

Extensive research has been done over the past few decades to determine if certain women run a higher risk of developing heart disease. A number of interesting medical studies have focused on a variety of factors that appear linked to the likelihood of developing heart disease. These include specific physical characteristics, family history, blood lipid profile, hypertension, diabetes, as well as lifestyle factors such as diet, smoking, lack of activity and stress.

Physical Characteristics

Age. As mentioned earlier, the older the woman, the greater her risk of developing heart disease. The highest incidence is in women older than age 65.

Body Weight. Women weighing 20 to 30 percent over their ideal weight are considered to be at greater risk of developing heart disease. This was noted in an eight-year study by Harvard Medical School, which followed more than 115,000 women. Excess weight was found to be a significant factor in women developing coronary artery disease during the study period.

Body Shape—Distribution of Fat. Not only is overall obesity a risk factor but also how the fat is distributed on the body. Women with excess weight concentrated in their midbody, with a shape like an apple, have a higher risk of coronary artery disease than pear-shaped women, who distribute their fat to their hips and thighs.

Family History of Heart Disease. You are at higher risk of developing heart disease if close relatives have had a heart attack at an early age. Statistically, the risk increases if your father had a heart attack before age 56 or your mother before age 60. Similarly, you are at higher risk if any of your grandparents had a heart attack at a young age.

Blood Lipid Profile

Elevated Triglycerides. Elevated triglycerides are a type of fat consisting of three fatty acid molecules hooked to a glycerol backbone. Triglycerides are the form in which fat is stored in the body's tissues. Normal triglyceride levels range from 50 to 200 mg/dl. Triglycerides elevated in the blood to a level of 200 mg/dl or greater indicate a greater risk of developing coronary artery disease.

Elevated Total Cholesterol and LDL Cholesterol. Cholesterol is a yellowish, waxy substance manufactured in the body primarily by the liver and to a lesser extent by the intestines. We also ingest cholesterol in our diet when we eat dairy and meat products and fish. Cholesterol is needed for the synthesis of our sex hormones; it is the initial ingredient for sex hormone production. Cholesterol is also necessary for the synthesis of cell membranes and other essential body substances such as the sheath or coating of the nerves and bile.

How effectively cholesterol is used depends on its efficient transport throughout the body and how well the body can store or dispose of any excess. Transportation in the body is a potential problem because the fatty cholesterol isn't soluble in blood, which is mostly water. To solve this problem the body packages the cholesterol with a protein that allows the fat to be mixed with the blood. This process takes place in the liver where several types of cholesterol-protein mixtures are produced.

The major type of cholesterol-protein manufactured is low-density lipoprotein, or LDL, the body's main carrier of cholesterol. When LDL levels are elevated, it is believed to remain in the blood stream. The excessive levels of LDL are thought to injure the endothelium (the inner lining of the blood vessel wall), thereby initiating plaque formation. Thus, LDL is considered to be the "bad" type of cholesterol. Women with a total blood cholesterol above 240 mg/dl and a LDL level above 160 mg/dl are thought to be at high risk of heart disease. For the greatest degree of protection, total cholesterol should be below 180 mg/dl and the LDL below 130 mg/dl.

Decreased HDL Cholesterol. The liver makes another type of lipoprotein called high-density lipoprotein, or HDL, the "good" type of cholesterol. This is because HDL picks up and carries excess cholesterol back to the liver where it is secreted into the bile. The bile empties the excess cholesterol into the intestinal tract where it is excreted from the body through bowel movements. When the HDL is less than 35 mg/dl, a woman is considered to be at high risk of coronary artery disease. The HDL is about 55 mg/dl in a lower risk woman.

Elevated LDL to HDL Ratio. The ratio between the LDL and HDL is also an important indicator of heart disease risk. Ideally, the LDL to HDL ratio should be no higher than 4:1. For example, if your LDL is 150 and HDL is 30, then your ratio is 5:1 which puts you in the high-risk category.

Hypertension

High blood pressure is a significant risk factor for developing coronary artery disease. Sixty million Americans have elevated blood pressure readings. Nearly half of these are women. Blood pressure is considered to be elevated when the reading is above 140/90. The first number indicates the systolic pressure, the pressure that occurs when the heart contracts and pushes blood through the arterial circulation. The second number indicates the diastolic blood pressure, the pressure in the arteries when the heart relaxes between beats. Not only does hypertension increase the likelihood of heart attacks, but it also increases your risk of strokes and kidney disease.

Diabetes

The Framingham Study, an important study of cardiovascular disease risk, found that women with diabetes have twice as high a risk of developing a heart attack as nondiabetic women. Diabetic women are also at higher risk of developing serious visual problems and kidney complications, as well as hypertension and higher cholesterol levels.

Lifestyle Factors

In the last decade, research has indicated that lifestyle factors play a major role in the development of disease. Life patterns such as diet, smoking, obesity, sedentary behavior and high stress all contribute to a high risk profile for heart disease and stroke.

Cigarette Smoking. Women smokers have an increased risk of heart attacks and strokes (as do men smokers). This is because smoking narrows the diameter of the blood vessels, impairing circulation. Smokers are also more likely to have higher levels of the bad LDL and lower levels of the good HDL.

Cigarette smoking is also considered a major cause of stroke, the third leading cause of death in the United States. Nicotine increases the heart rate, which in turn, raises the blood pressure. Hypertension can be a precursor to stroke.

Unfortunately, 27 percent of all women smoke, and this percentage is not declining rapidly despite the great amount of public information on the health perils of smoking. Women smokers also enter menopause two to three years earlier than nonsmokers.

Physical Inactivity. Women with sedentary lifestyles have a three times higher risk of developing heart disease than women who are physically active. The heart is a muscle that needs to be exercised. Women who engage in aerobic exercise such as walking at least three times a week for a half hour have a lower resting heart rate, greater lung capacity, and an improved ability to handle stress.

Stress. Several studies suggest that severe stress is a risk factor in women for developing coronary artery disease. Unfortunately, women have not been studied as frequently as men. Many studies have been done on the Type A hard-driving, aggressive male personality. However, women with multiple home and work responsibilities are often as hard driving and stressed as men. This can, over time, predispose certain women to an increased risk of heart attack.

Diet. In 1989 the National Research Council reported evidence of a direct relationship between dietary fat intake and the risk of cardiovascular disease, cancer and stroke. You can limit your long-term risk of developing these conditions by 20 percent if you limit your fats to 30 percent of your daily calories, keep saturated fats to less than 10 percent and keep cholesterol levels down.

Female-related Risk Factors

Some risk factors for heart disease are particularly female and directly relate to menopause and hormone levels.

Menopausal Status. The risk of coronary artery disease increases two to three fold once a woman enters natural menopause. Research studies, including the Framingham Study (which has been ongoing since 1949), have confirmed that premenopausal women with intact ovarian function enjoy significant protection against the development of heart attacks.

Surgical or Natural Menopause Before Age 45. Recent studies have shown that women who undergo a hysterectomy with removal of their ovaries during the premenopausal years have three times more risk of coronary artery disease than women who cease menstruating later. Similarly, a study of 122,000 nurses found that women who went through surgical menopause before age 35 have two to seven times the risk of heart attack; the risk is also higher in women who go through natural menopause at an early age. Estrogen appears to confer significant protection against heart attacks during a woman's active reproductive years. The longer a woman menstruates, the more years of estrogenic protection her vascular system enjoys.

Hormonal Therapy for Heart Disease Prevention

The effects of estrogen alone and of combined estrogen-progestin therapy have been studied for the effects on the cardiovascular system. HRT has been primarily studied in two different ways: looking at the effects of hormonal therapy on cardiovascular disease risk factors and assessing the incidence of cardiovascular disease in women using HRT compared with control women.

Estrogen Therapy

The use of ERT alone has been found to have beneficial effect on blood lipid patterns, a major factor for cardiovascular disease. Estrogen does improve the lipoprotein profile. It increases the level of HDL, the "good" cholesterol, and decreases the level of LDL, the "bad" cholesterol linked to coronary artery disease. It is estimated that 50 percent of the protective effect of estrogen on the cardiovascular system is due to estrogen's effect on lipoproteins. The balance of the protection is due to the direct effect of estrogen on the blood vessels and blood cells. Estrogen has a relaxant effect on blood vessels and improves arterial blood flow throughout the body. This benefits blood flow to the heart through its effect on the coronary arteries.

Even with all of these positive influences on the cardiovascular system, ERT does have one negative side effect. Its use can cause a moderate increase in the triglyceride level. As mentioned earlier, elevated triglycerides are a minor risk factor for the development of heart disease. However, on balance, given the mostly positive effects that ERT has on blood lipids, many physicians prescribe ERT to women for its long-term cardiovascular benefits. ERT prescribed for postmenopausal use does not appear to significantly affect blood pressure, carbohydrate metabolism, or blood coagulation.

The clinical benefits of ERT are noted in a number of research studies. According to one study done by Dr. Trudy Bush and her colleagues through the National Institute of Health, the death rate from heart disease was only one-third as high in women on ERT as in a control group of women not on estrogen. Another study of 2,000 women over an eight year period from the Lipid Research Clinics found that the death rate from cardiovascular disease was significantly lower when women used ERT than it was for the control group of women. Other research has found that not only does ERT protect women from death due to heart attacks, but it also appears to reduce the likelihood of developing a heart attack by 50 percent. The most significant study to date, published in the *New England Journal of Medicine* in September 1991, indicated that the heart benefits of estrogen far outweigh any risks. Almost 50,000 nurses were studied for ten years, and the results showed that those taking estrogen after menopause were half as likely to develop or die from cardiovascular disease. This protection appears to extend to women who have undergone surgical menopause and use ERT.

Not all studies, however, agree with these findings. One study published in *The New England Journal of Medicine* in 1985 concluded that estrogen increases the risk of heart attack. An earlier study in 1978 found an increased risk of cardiovascular disease in women using estrogen who smoked cigarettes. However, following the published results of the Nurses Health Study, the largest and most carefully controlled study of estrogen and heart disease, the conclusion is that the benefits of estrogen far outweigh any risks. Therefore, the consensus seems to be toward the protective action of ERT against cardiovascular disease.

Estrogen-Progestin Therapy

Although estrogen alone has been studied for its effects on the cardiovascular system, this does not mirror the type of HRT that most postmenopausal women use. Most physicians prescribe combined estrogen and progestin therapy to women who have an intact uterus. As mentioned earlier, this is done to prevent the likelihood of developing endometrial cancer. This has concerned both physicians and researchers because progesterone has the opposite effect on blood lipids that estrogen does. Progesterone increases LDL and decreases HDL. As a result, a concern is that the addition of progestins, although necessary for protection against uterine cancer, would negate the beneficial effects of estrogen on the cardiovascular system. Several studies have been done to compare the risks and benefits of estrogen alone versus estrogen-progestin therapy. To date, studies lasting more than 12 months do not suggest that progestins used in HRT affect blood lipids adversely. Early studies suggest that oral micronized progesterone may have even fewer adverse side effects than the synthetic form of progesterone commonly used. However, much more research remains to be done in this area.

Estrogen Therapy for Stroke Prevention

Every year 86,000 women die of strokes. Another effect of estrogen may be to reduce the incidence of strokes.

Stroke is a sudden and severe loss of blood flow in the brain caused by a blocked vessel. This condition may be caused by hemorrhage, thrombosis or a clot and is associated with hypertension. The medical term for stoke is cerebral vascular accident or CVA. The event may result in tragic, often irreversible brain damage. Small strokes may cause dementia, also an irreversible condition.

While some estrogen studies have shown no protective effects against stroke, current research appears to support the theory that using estrogen results in fewer strokes. A 1993 study published in the *Archives of Internal Medicine* of almost 2,000 white postmenopausal women found that when women used estrogen, they had fewer strokes (31 percent reduction) and when strokes did occur, they were less likely to die (63 percent reduction in deaths from strokes).

In 1991, over 8,000 women in a retirement home in California were monitored. Those still taking ERT after at least 15 years on the medication suffered 40 percent fewer deaths from heart disease and stroke than those who had never used estrogen. Finally, in the article, *Cardiovascular Health and Disease in Women*, it was noted that postmenopausal ERT does not increase the risk of heart disease or stroke even among women who had a prior CVA or who have hypertension.

Even with all the benefits that ERT and HRT can confer on total cardiovascular risk, the decrease in incidence is only 50 percent. To significantly reduce your risk, it is important to combine HRT with healthy lifestyle practices and prevention, a low-fat, high-nutrient diet, avoidance of cigarette smoking and an active exercise program. And for some of you, practice relaxation techniques and learn to manage stress better to further reduce your risk. HRT plus a healthy, preventive lifestyle can provide optimal levels of cardiovascular disease protection against a heart attack or stroke.

General Risk Factors for Coronary Artery Disease

Physical characteristics
> Age
> Body weight
> Body shape—distribution of fat

Family history of heart disease

Blood lipid profile
> Elevated triglycerides
> Elevated total cholesterol and LDL cholesterol
> Decreased HDL cholesterol
> Elevated LDL to HDL ratio

Hypertension

Diabetes Mellitus

Lifestyle factors
> Cigarette smoking
> Physical inactivity
> Stress

Female-related risk factors
> Menopausal status
> Surgical or natural menopause before age 45

Alternatives to Hormone Replacement Therapy

❖ ❖ ❖

10

Dietary Principles
for Menopause Relief

$\mathcal{D}$iet plays a very important role in determining the health of menopausal women. The foods you choose may trigger hot flashes and other unpleasant menopausal symptoms, as well as increase your risk of developing such serious diseases as heart attacks, strokes, cancer and arthritis. On the other hand, foods chosen wisely for their high nutrient content and easy digestibility can decrease and even prevent symptoms of menopause.

The traditional American diet tends to work against us, because it is laden with unhealthy fat, sugar, salt and stimulants. If you follow this diet without making modifications as your body ages, your health will suffer. To change your eating habits in ways that will help create optimal health and wellbeing during your menopausal years requires knowledge about modern concepts of nutrition. Important research about how nutrition benefits the body has been on-going during the past 40 years, but very little of it has actually reached the consumer.

This chapter contains essential information about diet that you may use to change your own habits toward optimal health. I have used these guidelines for nearly 20 years. My patients have been delighted with the beneficial results. The first section discusses the foods that you should emphasize for good health. In the second section, I will provide information on which foods to avoid or limit.

Foods That Ease Menopausal Symptoms

This diet emphasizes high-nutrient foods such as beans and peas (legumes), whole grains, foods containing essential and healthy oils (including raw seeds and nuts), certain fish, and lots of fresh fruits and vegetables. There is evidence that this dietary approach can help relieve and prevent symptoms of menopause. These types of foods predominate in the traditional diets of many Asian and African cultures. Interestingly, menopausal symptoms tend to be much less prevalent and severe in these cultures. For example, these symptoms occur in 10 to 15 percent of Japanese women at midlife, in contrast with 80 to 85 percent of American women. Diet is thought to play a major role in the different ways women experience menopausal symptoms. Let us look at the benefits each of the healthy foods can bring you during your midlife years.

Beans and Peas (Legumes)

Soybean-based products actually help reduce and prevent menopausal symptoms. Soybeans are loaded with natural plant or phytoestrogens, called bioflavonoids. Japanese eat a lot of soybeans, so this may be one reason that the women report fewer menopausal problems. Certain bioflavonoids are weak estrogens, having 1/50,000 the potency of stilbestrol, a synthetic estrogen used in medical therapy several decades ago. As weak estrogens, these compounds bind to estrogen receptors and act as a substitute form of estrogen in the body. Although menopausal women are deficient in estrogen, the bioflavonoids can help reduce symptoms. In addition, bioflavonoid-containing foods may also have an anticarcinogenic effect, which could explain the lower incidence of breast cancer among Japanese women and lower mortality from prostate cancer among Japanese men.

Dietary studies show that men, women and children in Japan, as well as Americans following a macrobiotic diet or vegetarian diet, excrete 100 to 1000 times more beneficial bioflavonoids in their urine than people in Finland and the United States who eat a meat- and dairy-based diet, which has a bioflavonoid content 80 percent lower than a vegetarian-based diet.

A recent study published in *The British Medical Journal* described how shifting the diet towards phytoestrogen-containing foods can change certain menopause indicators. In this study, 25 menopausal women (average age of 59) were asked to supplement their normal diet with phytoestrogen-containing foods such as soy flour, flax seed oil and red clover sprouts. The women consumed these foods over a six-week period. Smears from the vaginal wall were taken every two weeks to see if the addition of estrogen-containing plant foods would cause a beneficial hormonal effect on the vagina. Typically, the vaginal mucosa thins out and becomes more prone to trauma and infections as the estrogen level drops with menopause. Interestingly, the vaginal mucosa responded significantly to the additional ingestion of soy flour and flax oil (although not to red clover sprouts), but returned to previous levels eight weeks after these foods were discontinued and the women went back to their usual diet.

In addition to the beneficial estrogenic effects of soybeans, legumes in general are excellent foods for menopausal women. Common sources include garbanzo beans, kidney beans, lima beans, black beans and lentils. All legumes are an excellent source of protein, particularly when combined with whole grains. When used together, the two foods provide the full range of essential amino acids, the building blocks of protein. In addition, legumes are an excellent source of fiber. The fiber content causes beans to be broken down and their nutrients, such as protein and carbohydrates, absorbed more slowly. This has many health benefits. The slow digestion of legume-based carbohydrates can help regulate the blood sugar level. As a result, legumes are an excellent food for women with blood sugar imbalances or diabetes. The fiber can help normalize bowel function and lower cholesterol levels by promoting excretion of cholesterol through the bowel movements.

Legumes are excellent sources of many other nutrients needed by menopausal women. These include calcium and magnesium, which are essential for strong bones and healthy muscle tone. Legumes also contain high levels of potassium, which help regulate the heart beat as well as provide muscle tone. Legumes are very high in iron, copper and zinc. Sufficient iron intake is particularly important for women with heavy menstrual bleeding who are beginning menopause. Legumes are also high in vitamin B-complex, essential for healthy liver function. The liver metabolizes estrogen so that it can be excreted efficiently from the body.

Whole Grains

Healthy grains for menopausal women include oats, corn, barley, millet, buckwheat, wild rice, brown rice and whole wheat. As with legumes, many whole grains are an excellent source of phytoestrogens. Whole grains contain lignins, a celluloselike material that provides structure to plants. Lignins, like bioflavonoids, have been found to be weakly estrogenic and can provide additional nutritional support to menopausal women deficient in this hormone. In addition, certain grainlike plants such as buckwheat are good sources of the bioflavonoid, rutin. This bioflavonoid is particularly helpful in its ability to strengthen capillaries and reduce heavy menstrual bleeding when women are just entering menopause. Bioflavonoids, along with vitamin C, have been used in medical studies to reduce heavy bleeding during this time, as well as when there is bleeding due to fibroid tumors and spontaneous abortions. One study of women who miscarried multiple pregnancies concluded that the bioflavonoid-vitamin C combination allowed 78 percent of high-risk women studied to carry their pregnancies to full term.

The high fiber content of whole grains also helps regulate estrogen levels because of the ability of fiber to bind estrogen in the intestinal tract and remove it from the body through bowel movements. As described earlier, estrogen circulates in the blood throughout the body, including the liver. The liver metabolizes estrogen from its more potent forms, estradiol and estrone, to a chemically inactive and weaker form, estriol. When the liver is functioning in a healthy manner, this occurs efficiently. The estrogen metabolites are then secreted into the bile and from there into the digestive tract. This whole process is called the enterohepatic circulation of estrogen.

A high-fat, low-fiber diet promotes the growth of certain bacteria in the intestinal tract that act chemically on these estrogen products. These bacteria convert the estrogen products back to estrone and estradiol, allowing reabsorption of the estrogen back into the body. As mentioned earlier in this book, estrone is the primary type of estrogen produced by the body after menopause and estradiol is the type of estrogen produced by the ovary during the active reproductive years. As a result of the intestinal bacteria, the levels of these two estrogens rise higher than estriol, their primary breakdown product. This abundance of the more potent forms of estrogen may not present a healthy estrogen profile. Research studies have shown that estradiol and estrone, as the more chemically active and potent forms of estrogen, may predispose women toward developing breast cancer, while estriol, a much weaker form of estrogen, may confer protection against breast cancer. Thus, a high-fiber, low-fat diet may help regulate not only the estrogen levels, but the types of estrogen circulating through a woman's body. A number of studies have shown that vegetarian women excrete two to three times more estrogen in their bowel movements than do women eating the typical high-fat, low-fiber diet.

Besides regulating estrogen levels, the high-fiber content of whole grains binds to cholesterol, increasing its excretion from the body through the digestive tract. This helps lower blood cholesterol levels, reducing a significant risk factor for heart attacks in postmenopausal women. The fiber in grain is very helpful in relieving constipation, as well as preventing other diseases of the digestive tract such as diverticulitis and hiatus hernia. Fiber may also have a protective effect against developing colon cancer, a disease also found more commonly in people who eat a high-fat, low-fiber diet.

Whole grains are excellent sources of carbohydrates capable of stabilizing blood sugar and helping eliminate sugar craving. They help prevent or control diabetes mellitus, a dangerous disease that predisposes people toward heart disease, blood vessel problems, infections and blindness. Fifty percent of our population over age 60 have blood sugar abnormalities, due in great part to the tremendous amount of high-sugared foods and sweets Americans eat. Whole grains, with their natural sweetness, can satisfy much of this craving in a healthful way.

In addition, whole grains are a major source of complete protein when combined in a meal with legumes. Whole grains also contain many excellent nutrients for menopausal women. They contain high levels of vitamin B and vitamin E, both of which are critical for healthy hormonal balance and regulating estrogen levels. This occurs through their beneficial effect on both the liver and ovaries. Whole grains' vitamin B and vitamin E content also help combat the fatigue and depression that can occur with the onset of menopause. Grains are high in magnesium which helps reduce muscle tension. They are also high in calcium, necessary for healthy bones and to relax muscle tension. Finally, whole grains are high in potassium. Potassium has a diuretic effect on body tissues and helps reduce bloating, which can be a problem for postmenopausal women.

Essential Fatty
Acid-Containing Foods

Healthy essential oils are extremely beneficial for menopausal women. Linoleic acid, which belongs to the Omega-6 family of fatty acids, is primarily found in raw seeds and nuts. Good sources include flax seed, pumpkin seeds, sesame seeds, sunflower seeds and walnuts. The other essential fatty acid, called linolenic acid, is a member of the Omega-3 family and is primarily found in certain fish such as trout, salmon, mackerel, as well as some plant sources like flax seeds, soy, pumpkin seeds, walnuts and green leafy vegetables. Both essential fatty acids must be derived from dietary sources because they cannot be produced by the body.

The body does not primarily burn the essential fatty acids for energy, unlike the saturated fats found in red meat, eggs, dairy products and a few plants such as palm and coconut oils. Instead, these fatty acids have special functions in the body necessary for good health and survival. The skin is full of fatty acids that, along with estrogen, provide moisture, softness and smooth texture. When the estrogen levels decline with menopause, moisture continues to be provided to the skin, vagina and bladder mucosa by increasing levels of fatty acid-containing foods. Flax seed oil is particularly good for dry skin because it contains high levels of both fatty acids. In addition, fatty acids are a main structural component of all cell membranes and are found in high levels in such important tissues as the brain and nerve cells, retina of the eye, adrenal gland and inner ear.

Besides relieving tissue dryness, essential fatty acids are also needed by the body as precursors for the production of important hormonelike chemicals called prostaglandins. There are over 30 types of prostaglandins manufactured by tissues throughout the body. The proper balance of prostaglandins can play a major role in relieving and preventing many diseases that occur predominantly in the postmenopausal period.

The series one prostaglandins are manufactured by the body from linoleic acid. These prostaglandins have many beneficial effects. One member of the series, called prostaglandin E, or PGE, is particularly helpful for menopausal women. It relaxes the blood vessels and improves circulation. It keeps the platelets, a component of blood, from sticking or clumping together. This reduces the likelihood of heart attacks and strokes by preventing blood clotting and obstruction of the blood vessels. Since the incidence of heart attacks increases ten-fold between the ages of 55 and 65, PGE can benefit women greatly.

In addition, PGE prevents inflammation, reducing the symptoms of arthritis. For many women, arthritis symptoms begin after they go through menopause. PGE also stimulates the immune system and helps insulin function effectively.

The series three prostaglandins are manufactured from the eicosapentaenoic acid (EPA) found in fish such as salmon and trout. They are also produced more slowly from plant sources containing linolenic acid. As mentioned earlier, flax oil is a particularly good food source of linolenic acid. One member of this series called PGE 3 has anticlotting effects similar to those of PGE. They also help reduce the likelihood of heart attacks and strokes when manufactured by the body in high levels. PGE 3 also decreases triglycerides levels, another risk factor for heart attacks. It also helps prevent the manufacture of PGE 2, an undesirable prostaglandin made from arachidonic acid, a fatty acid derived primarily from dietary sources of red meat and dairy products. Unlike PGE and PGE 3, arachidonic acid-derived PGE 2 actually promotes platelet aggregation or clumping, thereby initiating potentially dangerous clot formation. It also causes inflammation and fluid retention, which can predispose postmenopausal women towards arthritis and high blood pressure. Thus, it is important to favor fish, seeds and nuts as sources of protein to promote production of the "good" prostaglandins.

Vegetables

Vegetables are excellent foods that come in a wide variety of flavors, colors and textures. They are important for health because they are extremely rich in many vitamins and minerals. Recent research in the past two decades has also emphasized their importance in protecting postmenopausal women from diseases such as heart attacks, strokes, cancer and immune system breakdown.

Vegetables high in vitamin A usually have a orange, red or dark green color. These include squash, sweet potatoes, pepper, carrots, kale and lettuce, as well as many other common foods. Unlike animal-based sources of vitamin A, which contain an oil-soluble form of this vitamin, plant sources contain a precursor form of vitamin A called beta carotene. Beta carotene is converted to vitamin A by the liver and intestines once ingested into the body. This form tends to be very safe and is found in high doses in many foods. For example, one glass of carrot juice or a sweet potato each contains 20,000 international units [IU] of beta carotene. Many people eat two to three times this amount in their daily diet.

Research shows that vitamin A will protect against cancer and immune system deficiency. Of particular interest to menopausal women are studies showing that vitamin A may protect against breast cancer. Other research studies suggest that a high intake of plant foods containing beta carotene protects against heart attacks in high-risk people.

Many vegetables are also high in vitamin C, which has a protective effect against heart attack, cancer and immune system problems. Vitamin C is particularly important for transition menopausal women because, along with iron and bioflavonoids, it can protect against excessive menopausal bleeding. Research studies also suggest that vitamin C may help protect women from developing cervical cancer as well as vitamin A does. Vitamin C is important for wound healing and healthy skin. Vegetables high in vitamin C include potatoes, pepper, peas, tomatoes, broccoli, brussels sprouts, cabbage, cauliflower, kale and parsley.

Vegetables contain many other important nutrients such as iron, magnesium and calcium that protect against osteoporosis, anemia and excessive menstrual bleeding. Leafy green vegetables, such as beet greens, collards and dandelion greens, are excellent sources of these important nutrients. Other vegetables also have health enhancing properties. Onions and garlic decrease the blood's clotting tendency and lower serum cholesterol, which can help decrease the incidence of stroke and heart attack. Studies indicate that ginger root, onions and mushrooms may have a similar effect. Certain mushrooms may even stimulate immune system function. Some vegetables such as kelp are high in iodine and trace minerals, essential for healthy thyroid function. Use kelp as a seasoning to sprinkle on vegetables and grains. Be sure to eat your vegetables raw or lightly steamed to preserve their nutrient value. Do not boil or overcook vegetables, because vitamins and minerals can be lost through improper preparation.

Fruit

Fruits are an exceptional source of bioflavonoids and vitamin C which helps to control excessive menstrual flow as well as provide the body with weak plant sources of estrogen. The inner peel and pulp of the citrus fruit is an excellent source of bioflavonoids and, in fact, is used for commercial production of bioflavonoid supplements. This is, unfortunately, the more bitter part of the fruit that many women discard, unaware of the health benefits the inner peel and pulp can provide. Also, the skin of grapes, cherries and many berries are rich sources of bioflavonoids. So, it is better to eat the whole fruit rather than just drink the juice.

Adequate potassium intake is necessary for good health, and fruits are very good food sources of potassium. Potassium helps lower high blood pressure and protects against heart disease; it also decreases bloating and fluid retention. Medical studies show that potassium is beneficial in reducing menopause-related fatigue. Fruits high in potassium include bananas, oranges, grapefruits, berries, peaches, apricots and melons. Fruits are also an excellent source of vitamin C, which provides important protection against cancer and infectious diseases as well as heart disease. Most whole fruits contain some vitamin C—berries, oranges and melons provide exceptionally high levels of this essential nutrient. Yellow- and orange-colored fruits such as papaya, persimmon, apricot and tangerine should be included in your diet because of their high vitamin C content.

Although fruit is high in sugar, the high fiber content of the whole fruit slows down digestion, curbs appetite and stabilizes the blood sugar level. The high fiber content of many fruits make them excellent foods for women who experience constipation. Pineapple and papaya also contain enzymes that help to break down protein, so they promote food digestive function and speed up bowel transit time.

Be aware that fruit juice does not contain the bulk or fiber of whole fruit, so it does not stabilize blood sugar or have beneficial effects on bowel function. Juice acts more like the simple sugars found in candy, so it should be used sparingly. The whole fruit retains the sweet flavor and makes a healthy substitute for candies, cookies, cakes and other highly sugared foods. Use it as a snack or dessert instead of cookies, candies, pastries or ice cream.

Foods to Avoid or Limit with Menopause

Diet can have a negative affect on your health as you go through and beyond menopause, if your food selection is poorly chosen. Foods described in this section either accentuate menopausal symptoms or add to the risk of developing diseases that increase in incidence during the postmenopausal period. These include heart disease, stroke, high blood pressure, cancer, arthritis and diabetes, to name only the most common ones.

Caffeine-containing Foods

Caffeine-containing foods include beverages such as coffee, black tea, cola drinks and chocolate. These foods are used almost universally in our culture, both as stimulants and as emotional "treats." Caffeine belongs to a class of chemicals called methylxanthines, central nervous stimulants that increase alertness and energy level. Many menopausal women use a caffeinated beverage on a regular basis to combat fatigue and provide a pick-up in the morning. Many women depend on caffeine to be able to function energetically on a daily basis. This practice may accelerate during menopause when fatigue is often worse due to poor sleep quality. Hot flashes and perspiration can recur throughout the night, leaving women depleted of energy and exhausted.

Unfortunately, there are many negatives to the use of caffeinated beverages, which negate their initial benefits. Caffeine is an addictive chemical and a person often requires large amounts to provide wakefulness and alertness. When stopping regular caffeine intake, many people find that they are even more fatigued and tired. Regular caffeine users who stop caffeine intake abruptly even experience uncomfortable withdrawal symptoms such as throbbing headaches and mood changes. Menopausal women may find that psychological symptoms such as anxiety, irritability and mood swings that can occur due to hormonal deficiency are increased with caffeine intake. In addition, caffeine has a diuretic effect and increases the loss from the body of many minerals and vitamins essential to health during the menopausal years. Loss of potassium, zinc, magnesium, vitamin B and vitamin C accelerates with caffeine intake. Coffee also reduces the absorption of iron and calcium from food and supplemental sources, particularly when used at mealtimes. For women who want to prevent osteoporosis and iron-deficiency anemia, this is a concern. Finally, caffeine use is linked to an increased incidence of nodules and tenderness in women with benign breast disease.

Postmenopausal women at high risk for a heart attack or stroke because of family tendency or blood fat profile may want to avoid caffeine. Caffeine increases blood cholesterol and triglyceride levels, risk factors for heart attacks. In addition, caffeine raises the blood pressure, another risk factor for heart attacks and strokes (hypertension becomes increasingly prevalent with age). Caffeine also causes the heart to beat faster and increases the excitability of the system that conducts electrical impulses through the heart. This can lead to irregular heartbeat in susceptible women.

Luckily, many substitutes are available for women who like either the taste of coffee or the pick-me-up that it produces. Water processed *decaffeinated coffee* is often the easiest substitute to start with for women who like the flavor of coffee. Coffee substitutes that are grain-based, such as *Pero, Postum* and *Cafix,* are even better and ginger tea can have a vitalizing and energetic effect.

Alcohol

Alcohol will intensify almost every type of menopausal symptom. As a result, I recommend that women with active symptoms limit their intake or avoid alcoholic beverages entirely. The list of symptoms of menopause affected by alcohol intake includes hot flashes and mood swings. Unlike caffeine, alcohol is a central nervous system depressant, so its intake can increase menopausal fatigue and depression. This is particularly pronounced in women with night sweats and insomnia whose sleep quality is already poor.

In addition, alcohol has a diuretic effect on the body. During our active reproductive years, estrogen helps keep the skin and other tissues plump by causing fluid and salt retention in the body. As our estrogen levels begin to wane, excessive intake of alcohol can further dehydrate the skin and tissues, including the vaginal and bladder mucosa. Alcohol's diuretic effect also causes the loss of excessive amounts of essential minerals through the urinary tract. These include minerals needed for healthy bones such as calcium, magnesium and zinc. Women who are addicted to alcohol may also have a negative calcium balance because of poor nutritional habits. Alcoholics often eat less calcium-rich food and ignore their intake of other essential nutrients, preferring the empty, nonnutritive calories of alcohol.

Alcohol irritates the liver. It is metabolized by the liver to a chemical called acetaldehyde, which is liver toxic. In addition, excessive alcohol cannot be metabolized to glucose or glycogen (the storage form of glucose). Instead, it is metabolized and stored in the liver as fat. Excessive fat deposition in the liver can eventually lead to scarring and cirrhosis. Excessive alcohol intake can also affect the liver's ability to metabolize estrogen and can elevate the body's blood estrogen levels, particularly of the more chemically active forms of estrogen.

On the positive side, alcohol in small amounts can be a pleasurable social beverage. When used in amounts not exceeding four ounces of wine, ten ounces of beer, or one ounce of hard liquor per day, it can have a pleasant relaxing effect. It makes us more sociable and enhances the taste of food. Small amounts of alcohol may also increase the high-density lipoproteins, a type of blood fat that protects people against heart attacks. However, for optimal health, I recommend using alcohol no more than once or twice a week; this is true for women in midlife with no obvious menopausal symptoms.

Sugar

Sugar is one of the most overused foods in the United States. It is primarily utilized as a sweetening agent in the form of sucrose, which most of us know as white, granular table sugar. Sugar is a main ingredient of cookies, cakes, soft drinks, candies, ice cream, cereals and many other foods. Many women are unaware of how prevalent it is in convenience foods such as salad dressings, catsup, relish, and even some prepackaged main courses in the supermarket. Foods sold in natural food stores are highly sugared, too, although with different types of sweeteners such as fructose, maple syrup and honey. As a result of this national sweet tooth, the average American eats more than 120 pounds of sugar per year.

This dietary sugar is eventually metabolized to its simplest form in the body called glucose. Glucose by itself is essential for all cellular processes, because it is the major source of fuel our cells use to generate energy. However, when the body is flooded with too much sugar, it becomes overwhelmed, cannot process the sugar effectively and overreacts by pumping out large amounts of insulin. This is the hormone that helps drive glucose into the cells where it can be used as energy. When too much insulin is secreted, the blood sugar level falls, and hypoglycemia can occur. With continued overuse of sugar, the pancreas eventually "wears out" and is no longer able to clear sugar from the blood circulation efficiently. The blood sugar level rises and diabetes mellitus is the result. This tendency toward diabetes or high blood sugar levels increases dramatically after menopause. Research studies show that more than 50 percent of Americans have blood sugar imbalances by age 65.

Excess sugar intake also depletes the body's reserve of B-complex vitamins and many essential minerals by increasing their rate of utilization and sugar metabolism. This can increase anxiety, irritability and nervous tension that many women feel as they transition into menopause. One research study even suggests that a diet high in sugar may impair liver function and affect the liver's ability to metabolize estrogen. Highly sugared foods also promote tooth decay and gum disease. Many women, however, are addicted to sugar and have a difficult time controlling their intake once they start eating sugary foods such as cookies and candy.

Because sugar is so deleterious to good health, menopausal women might consider avoiding sugar entirely or limiting its use to small amounts on social occasions. Sugar can be easily substituted in recipes by using fruit, sugar substitutes like aspartame (if you can tolerate them without side effects—many women are sensitive to aspartame) or smaller amounts of more concentrated sweeteners. Also, become a label reader. If canned and bottled foods such as salad dressings, soft drinks or baked beans have sugar near the top of the list, the product probably contains too much sugar. Search out alternatives that don't contain sugar or items using it in very small amounts. If you crave sweets, keep fresh or dried fruits handy such as apples, bananas or dried figs. Whole fruit should satisfy your craving for sweets and has the added benefit of being high in many essential nutrients.

Salt

Condiments and food additives such as table salt and monosodium glutamate (MSG) generally contain large amounts of sodium. Sodium is one of the body's major minerals. Primarily found in the body's extracellular compartment in conjunction with potassium, the primary intracellular mineral, sodium helps regulate water balance in the cells. Water tends to accumulate where sodium is prevalent. Thus, an overabundance of sodium relative to the body's potassium levels can lead to edema, bloating and sometimes high blood pressure. These problems are very common in menopausal women who are increasingly at risk for developing cardiovascular problems with age. In addition, fluid retention often adds to excess pounds that can be so irksome to women after menopause. Many women complain that they gain 10 to 15 pounds after menopause and that the weight is very difficult to lose, even with dieting and exercise. Of even greater concern is the fact that excess sodium is a risk factor for osteoporosis because it accelerates calcium loss from the body.

Unfortunately, as with sugar, salt is prevalent in the American diet. In fact, salt and sugar are often found together in large amounts in frozen and canned foods, cheeses, potato chips, hamburgers, hot dogs, cured meats, pizzas and other common foods. Many of us eat so much salt (far beyond the recommended 2000 mg or 1 teaspoon per day) that our palates have become jaded. Many people feel that food tastes too bland without the addition of salt.

Luckily, many other available seasoning options are much better for your health. For flavoring, use garlic, basil, oregano and other herbs. Fresh foods such as vegetables, grains, legumes and meat contain all the salt we need, so added table salt isn't necessary. As for sugar, read the labels before you buy bottled, canned or frozen food. Don't buy a product if salt is listed as a main ingredient (near the top of the list). Many brands in the health food stores and supermarkets now distribute foods labeled "no salt added" or "reduced salt content." Be sure to buy these rather than the high-salt content foods. Also, eat plenty of fresh fruits and vegetables because they are excellent sources of potassium and other essential nutrients. Potassium helps balance the sodium in the body and regulate the blood pressure to keep it at normal levels.

Meat, Dairy Products and Saturated Oils

At first glance, it may not be apparent that meat, dairy products and saturated oils have much in common. However, they are the main sources of fat in the typical American diet. Unlike the healthy fats that were described in the preceding section (found primarily in vegetable sources such as raw seeds and nuts, leafy green vegetables and fish), these fats are derived from saturated fat sources. When used in excess, they contribute to such common health problems as heart disease, cancer, obesity and arthritis. Unfortunately, 40 percent (rather than the ideal 20-25 percent) of the calories in the American diet come from unhealthy, meat-derived saturated fats.

Saturated fat tends to increase the cholesterol levels in the blood, particularly the high-risk, low-density lipoproteins that initiate the plaque formation in the blood vessels. Plaque formation can eventually lead to heart attacks and strokes. In contrast, the "good" fats derived from fish and vegetable sources can prevent heart attacks by reducing the tendency for the blood to clot. A high-saturated-fat diet can also lead to obesity in women of all ages. Menopausal women are particularly at risk because their metabolism slows down with age and they burn calories less efficiently. One gram of fat contains nine calories versus the four calories contained in one gram of protein or carbohydrate. As a result, fatty foods are much higher in calories per unit weight. Although saturated fats do provide the body with a concentrated source of energy, very few of us need these extra calories. Instead of burning the fat for energy, we tend to store it in our cells as excess poundage.

As mentioned earlier, a high-fat, low-fiber diet is also associated with colon cancer, prostate cancer in men, and some breast cancer in women. A high-fat diet promotes the conversion of estrogen metabolites by anaerobic bacteria in the intestinal tract to forms of estrogen that can be easily reabsorbed back into the body. This elevates the blood estrogen level with types of estrogen that may increase the susceptibility to breast cancer in certain women. In contrast, lowering the amount of dietary fat while increasing the amount of high fiber foods in the diet can help reduce the risk of hormone-dependent cancers in women.

Many American women base their meals on meat and dairy entrees like steaks, chops, oversized meat sandwiches, cheese sandwiches and yogurt. Unfortunately, large amounts of meat-based protein can increase the risk of osteoporosis. Meat protein is acidic; when a woman eats meat in excessive amounts, her body must buffer the acid load that meat creates. One way the body accomplishes this is by dissolving the bones. The calcium and other minerals released from the bones help restore the body's acid-alkaline balance. (This process does not occur with dairy products, which already contain calcium.) One study comparing the incidence of osteoporosis in meat-eating women (omnivores) with that in vegetarians found a dramatic difference in bone density after age 60. Between the ages of 60 and 89, vegetarian women lost 18 percent of their bone mass, but meat-eating women lost 35 percent of their bone mass—quite a striking difference. Other studies show that the amount of protein eaten will make a difference in actual calcium levels; protein intake over three ounces a day causes loss of the calcium from the urinary tract. This has been found to be true even in low-risk groups such as young, healthy males.

Finally, meat, dairy products and saturated oils (such as coconut and palm-kernel oil) are difficult to digest. As women age, they secrete less hydrochloric acid and fewer of the digestive enzymes needed for fat and protein breakdown in the intestinal tract. In one study, 40 percent of postmenopausal women lacked hydrochloric acid. Without sufficient hydrochloric acid, meat and other sources of protein are difficult to break down and thus, cannot be utilized properly by the body. In addition, calcium and iron absorption becomes more difficult without sufficient stomach acid.

Women who are concerned about eliminating dairy products from their diet because dairy foods are great sources of calcium can choose many other good food sources of calcium. These include beans and peas, raw seeds and nuts, green leafy vegetables, canned salmon, broccoli, parsley and blackstrap molasses. Using a daily calcium supplement is probably a good idea because you are assured of receiving an optimal amount of calcium, whether your diet is fortified or not.

For optimal protein intake, your diet should emphasize whole grains, beans and peas, seeds, nuts and fish high in the beneficial Omega-3 fatty acids. It is best to eliminate red meat and dairy products or use them occasionally in small portions. A truly optimal diet for the postmenopausal woman is one with high-nutrient content, low-stress foods and easy digestibility.

Summary Chart
Foods for Menopause Relief

Beans and peas (legumes)
Whole grains
Essential fats
   Raw seeds and nuts
   Green leafy vegetables
   Fish
Vegetables
Fruits

Summary Chart
Foods to Limit or Avoid

Caffeine-containing foods

    Coffee

    Black tea

    Cola drinks

    Chocolate

Alcohol

Sugar

Salt

Meat, dairy products and saturated oils

11

Menus, Meal Plans & Recipes

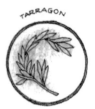

*P*roper meal planning is very important if your goal is to use dietary measures to relieve and prevent menopausal symptoms without the use of estrogen replacement therapy. However, even if you are currently using hormonal therapy, a good menopause-relief diet should be followed for its general health benefits. The high-nutrient content of meals designed for menopause relief, as well as their lack of high-stress ingredients such as saturated fats and sugar, helps prevent many of the diseases that become increasingly common after midlife, such as heart disease, cancer, arthritis and diabetes mellitus.

As mentioned in the previous chapter, menopausal symptoms are much less common and tend to be milder in intensity in countries outside the United States; for example, the Japanese follow dietary practices that are quite different from the American diet. Societies with a low incidence of menopausal symptoms tend to eat a diet based on vegetable protein or fish with lots of unrefined fiber. In contrast, the American diet is based on the use of milk, egg and meat protein as well as refined flour, sugar and other stressful ingredients. These foods are usually favored over whole fruits, vegetables, grains and other highly nutritious foods.

While you do not have to eat foods from other cultures (which might taste strange and unfamiliar) to be free of menopausal symptoms, some simple dietary modifications will make a major difference in your health. In this chapter I have included many helpful menopause-relieving menus and recipes you can add to your roster. Over the years, these meal planning guidelines have helped many of my patients implement their own self-help programs. Their feedback has been very positive. Many patients have noted an immediate difference in their health and well-being and found the new foods delicious and satisfying. I hope these dietary suggestions will be helpful to you, too.

General Guidelines

Before discussing the actual meal plans, consider three principles that make the transition process easier.

Make Dietary Changes Gradually

Make the transition to a healthful menopause-relief diet in an easy and nonstressful manner. Don't try to change all your dietary habits at one time by making a clean sweep of your refrigerator and pantry. Instead, substitute several healthy foods for high-stress foods you have been eating. To do this, periodically review the lists of foods to limit and those to emphasize. Each time you review this list, pick several foods you are willing to eliminate and several to try. Review these lists as often as you choose, but try to do it on a regular basis. Every small change you make in your diet will help.

Simple and Easy-to-Prepare Meals

Many women lead busy, active lives and don't have time to cook complicated meals. For that reason, my meal plans are quick and simple to prepare, with the main emphasis on foods that are delicious and high in nutrition. For those who are accustomed to eating quick meals at fast-food restaurants or commercial snack food that is high in fat, sugar and food additives, these simple meals offer a much healthier alternative.

Guidelines for Your Own Creations

Use these menus and recipes as a starting point to create your own meal plans and food combinations. Adapt your favorite dishes using the ideas contained in this chapter so that your meals are healthful rather than harmful.

Breakfast Menus

Breakfast is the most important meal of the day. Unfortunately, many women skip breakfast entirely, which can increase menopause-related fatigue, nervousness and mood swings. Other women fall into the American habit of grabbing fast foods in the morning. They eat doughnuts, sweet rolls and coffee in hopes of getting quick energy; instead, these foods can increase menopause-related nervous tension and irritability. Others may eat hearty breakfasts full of high-stress foods—eggs, bacon, milk, toast and butter. The high fat and salt content of these foods further stress the body and impair your health.

The healthy breakfast plan includes beverages, fruits and whole-grain foods. It also contains essential fatty acids and phytoestrogens such as flax seed and soy products.

Luckily, breakfast has been one of the easiest meals for my patients to restructure along healthier lines. You probably eat breakfast at home alone or with family members. It tends to be a smaller and simpler meal. You may want to make healthy dietary changes in your breakfast first and then move on to lunch and dinner.

The easy-to-prepare menus in this section provide a variety of healthful and delicious breakfast meals. They can also act as guidelines for you to create your own meal plans. Recipes for foods marked with an asterisk are included later in this chapter.

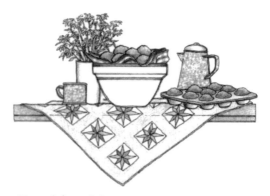

Breakfast Menus

Flax shake*
Rice cakes with sesame-tofu
   spread*

Nondairy milk breakfast shake
Bran muffin

Instant flax cereal
Peppermint tea

Tofu cereal*
Rose hip tea

Millet cereal*
Melon
Spring water

Oatmeal cereal #2*
Banana
Roasted grain beverage
   (coffee substitute)

Oatmeal cereal #1
Chamomile tea

Whole grain toast
Sesame-tofu spread*
Apple
Mint tea

Corn muffin with flax oil
Strawberries
Orange juice

Rice cakes
Raw sesame butter and
   fruit preserves
Sliced grapefruit
Spring water

Lunch and Dinner Menus

These lunch and dinner menus give you a variety of ways to organize your meals. A healthy menopause program combines a variety of soups, salads, sandwiches, fresh fruits, vegetables, legumes (beans and peas) and starches, as well as one-dish combination plates, and preferably fish if meat protein is to be used. If you include poultry and red meat in your meals, these items should be used in small amounts, preferably as a garnish for a vegetarian-based meal. Try the meals in this section instead of the heavy meat- and cheese-centered dishes that form the nucleus of so many fast foods and deli offerings. They are high in unhealthy saturated fats, salt and excessive calories.

Soup Menus

Lentil-tofu-rice soup*
Tomato and cucumber salad
Whole grain bread

Split pea-tofu soup*
Cole slaw
Applesauce

Vegetable soup
Tuna sandwich
Apple slices

Creamy carrot soup*
Broccoli with lemon*
Baked potato and flax oil*
Banana

Tomato soup
Kasha*
Rye bread with flax oil
Banana

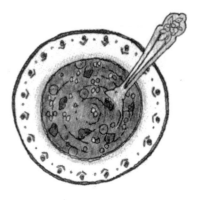

One-Dish
Vegetarian Meals

Pasta with flax oil and garlic*
Mixed green salad

Vegetarian tacos*
Low-salt salsa

Tofu and almond stir fry*
Steamed rice

Two-bean dish*
Romaine lettuce salad
Whole grain bread

Hummus and tahini*
Rye bread
Raw carrot and celery sticks

Rice and tofu tabouli
Black olives
Sliced tomatoes

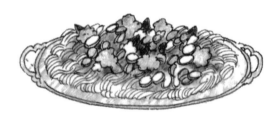

Salad Meals

Spinach salad
Corn muffins and flax oil

Beet salad
Rye bread with flax spread*

Tofu-wild rice salad*
Sliced tomatoes

Brown rice and tofu salad*
Apple and banana slices

Apple and walnut salad
Rice cakes with
    sesame-tofu spread*

Fish Meals

Poached salmon*
Brown rice
Steamed carrots*

Broiled trout*
Baked potato with flax oil*
Steamed artichoke

Broiled tuna
Mixed green salad
Broccoli with lemon*

Broiled sole with lemon
Sliced tomatoes and cucumber
Steamed red potatoes
Green beans and almonds*

Grilled halibut
Brown rice
Green beans and almonds*
Cole slaw

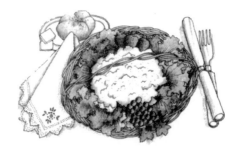

Recipes

4 tablespoons raw flax seeds
2 bananas
6 ounces water
6 ounces apple juice
1 tablespoon of vegetarian
    (soy- or rice-based) protein
    powder

Flax Shake   *Serves 2*
Grind flax seeds to a powder
using a coffee or seed grinder.
Place the powdered flax seeds
in a blender. Add the remaining ingredients and blend.
This recipe is high in essential
fatty acids, calcium, magnesium and potassium, necessary
for healthy bones and heart
function, as well as stabilizing
one's mood.

Non-Dairy Milk
Breakfast Shake *Serves 2*

2 cups nondairy milk (soy or
    other base)
2 ounces soft tofu
3 tablespoons flax oil
1 large banana
3/4 cup berries (strawberries,
    boysenberries, blueberries
    or raspberries)

Combine all ingredients in a
blender. Blend until smooth and
serve. This delicious, creamy
shake is high in essential fatty
acids, phytoestrogens, vitamin C
and calcium, all important nutrients for menopausal women.

Instant Flax Cereal

4 tablespoons raw flax seeds
4–8 ounces nondairy vanilla
    milk (soy or other base)
1/2 banana, sliced
sweetener (to taste)

Grind raw flax seeds into a powder using a seed or coffee grinder.
Place powder in a cereal bowl
and slowly add the nondairy
milk, stirring the mixture together.
The flax mixture will thicken into
a texture like cream of rice or
oatmeal. Top the cereal with
sliced bananas. Add sweetener
if desired. Eat the mixture right
away; flax seeds are sensitive to
light, air and temperature. This
cereal should be eaten cold, without cooking.

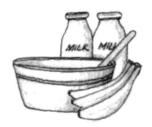

Tofu Cereal
Serves 2

4 ounces soft tofu
2 ounces nondairy vanilla milk
2 tablespoons flax oil
1 banana
1 apple
15 raw almonds
sweetener (if desired)

Combine all ingredients in a food processor. Blend until creamy. Pour into a bowl and serve. This is a helpful cereal for menopausal women, high in essential fatty acids, calcium, magnesium and potassium.

Millet Cereal
Serves 2

1 cup millet
2 cups water
1 teaspoon canola oil
4 ounces nondairy milk, vanilla
   (soy or other base)
1 tablespoon honey
1 tablespoon raw sunflower
   seeds
1 tablespoon raw sesame seeds

Wash millet with cold water. Combine millet, water and canola oil in a pot and bring to a boil. Turn heat to low, cover and cook without stirring about 25 to 35 minutes, until millet is soft. Don't check before 20 minutes, since this lets out too much stream. Fluff up the millet and spoon into serving bowls. Add the remaining ingredients. Mix and serve. Raw sunflower and sesame seeds are excellent sources of essential fatty acids, calcium, magnesium and potassium, important nutrients for menopausal women.

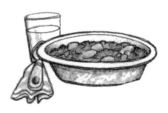

2/3 cup oats
1-1/2 cups water
2 tablespoons ground, raw
flax seeds
2-4 ounces nondairy milk,
vanilla flavored
1/2 banana
2 teaspoons honey

Oatmeal Cereal #1 *Serves 2*

Boil water in a pot. Stir in oats and return to a boil. Reduce heat to medium-low. Cook uncovered for 5 minutes, stirring occasionally. Remove from heat; let stand a few minutes. Stir in ground raw flax seeds followed by nondairy milk and honey. Serve.

2/3 cup oats
1-1/2 cups water
3 tablespoons flax oil
2 teaspoons maple syrup

Oatmeal Cereal #2 *Serves 2*

Boil water in a pot; stir in oats. Return mixture to a boil; reduce heat to medium-low. Cook uncovered for 5 minutes, stirring occasionally. Remove from heat and let stand for a few minutes. Stir in flax oil and maple syrup. Serve.

4 tablespoons raw flax seeds
1/2 lemon, juiced
1/2 teaspoons Bragg's Liquid
Amino Acids
2 tablespoon of water

Flax Spread *Serves 4*

Grind the flax seeds to a powder using a coffee or seed grinder. Add the remaining ingredients and mix into a paste. Use as a spread with rice cakes or crackers.

1/4 cup soft tofu
3/8 cup raw sesame butter
1/4 cup honey

Sesame-Tofu
Spread *Makes 1-1/2 cups*

Combine all ingredients in a blender. Use as a spread with rice cakes or crackers.

Split Pea-Tofu Soup   *Serves 4*

1 cup split peas
1/2 cup diced firm tofu
1/2 onion, chopped
1 small carrot, sliced
1 quart water
1/4 to 1/2 teaspoons sea salt
  or salt substitute

Wash peas. Place peas, onion and carrot in a pot. Add the water. Bring to a boil, then turn heat to low and cover pot. Cook for 45 minutes. Add sea salt and tofu. Continue to cook until peas are soft. Soup may be cooled and then pureed in a blender if you prefer a creamy texture.

Lentil-Tofu-Rice Soup   *Serves 4*

1 cup lentils
1/2 cup diced firm tofu
1/2 cup cooked brown rice
1/2 onion, chopped
1/2 cup carrots, chopped
1 to 1-1/2 quarts water
1 teaspoon brown rice miso

Wash lentils. Place lentils, onion, carrots, water and miso in a pot. Bring to a boil, then turn heat to low, cover pot and simmer for 45 minutes or until lentils are soft. Vary the amount of water depending on the desired thickness of the soup.

Creamy Carrot Soup   *Serves 4*

4 cups carrots, peeled and
  sliced
1-1/4 cups onions, diced
1/2 cup sweet red pepper
4 cups vegetable broth
1-1/2 tablespoons ginger
  root, grated
1-1/2 cup nondairy milk,
  vanilla flavored (soy or
  other base)

Combine carrots, onions, red peppers, vegetable broth and ginger in a large pot; cook for a half hour or until carrots are tender. Strain the vegetables and puree in a food processor. Add broth and non-dairy milk to blender and puree together. Return soup to cooking pot. Cook on low for five minutes. Serve.

Tofu-Wild Rice Salad   *Serves 4*

6 ounces tofu
2 cups cooked wild rice
3 scallions, chopped
1/4 to 1/2 cup minced parsley
1/2 green pepper, minced
herbal oil and vinegar dressing

Cut tofu into bite-size pieces. Combine with all the other ingredients in a bowl. Mix with your favorite herbal oil-and-vinegar dressing to taste. Note: Brown rice may be substituted for wild rice.

Brown Rice and Tofu Salad   *Serves 4*

2 cups cooked brown rice
4 ounces diced firm tofu
1 green onion, diced
1/4 cup raisins
1-1/2 ounces blanched almonds
1/4 cup peas, cooked
1/4 cup green pepper
1/4 cup celery

Combine all ingredients in a bowl. The salad may be dressed with a vinaigrette dressing or with a dressing made by combining 1-1/2 tablespoons seasoned rice wine vinegar, 1/2 teaspoon Worcestershire sauce, and 2-1/2 tablespoons mayonnaise.

Kasha   *Serves 4*

1 cup kasha (buckwheat groats)
3-1/4 cups water
pinch sea salt

Bring ingredients to a boil, lower heat and simmer for 25 minutes or until soft. The grains should be fluffy like rice. Buckwheat is an excellent source of bioflavonoids, an important phytoestrogen for menopausal women.

4 sweet potatoes
1 tablespoon canola oil
1 tablespoon flax oil for
each potato

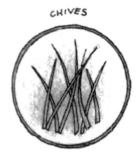

CHIVES

4 russet or Idaho potatoes
1 tablespoon vegetable oil
1 tablespoon flax oil for
each potato

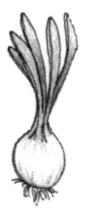

Baked Sweet Potato   *Serves 4*

Preheat oven to 400°F. Wash the potatoes then rub with canola oil. Bake for 45 to 60 minutes, or until soft when pierced with a fork. Garnish with flax oil. Honey, maple syrup or chopped raw pecans may also be used. Sweet potatoes are an excellent source of beta carotene. A diet high in beta carotene-containing foods helps reduce the incidence of breast cancer.

Baked Potato   *Serves 4*

Preheat oven to 400°F. Wash the potatoes, rub them with vegetable oil and bake for 45 to 60 minutes or until soft when pierced with a fork. Garnish with flax oil. Other garnishes can include chopped green onions or soy cheese. Potatoes are an excellent food taste-wise to use with essential fatty acids like flax oil. They are also easy to digest and good sources of nutrients like vitamin C.

Steamed Kale
Serves 4

1 bunch kale (stems removed), chopped
juice of 1 lemon
2-3 tablespoons olive oil
pinch of sea salt

Steam the kale until tender. Dress with lemon juice, olive oil and sea salt. Kale is an excellent source of calcium for menopausal women, since the calcium contained in kale absorbs and assimilates well.

Broccoli with Lemon
Serves 4

1 pound broccoli
1/2 lemon, juiced
4 tablespoons flax oil

Cut the broccoli into small flowerets; steam for 6 minutes or until tender. Squeeze lemon juice over broccoli and add the flax oil. Mix and serve. For an exciting taste treat try substituting Bragg's Liquid Amino Acids for the juiced lemon. Broccoli is a good source of calcium and magnesium, important nutrients for healthy bones. It is also high in vitamin A and other nutrients thought to confer protection against cancer.

Steamed Carrots
Serves 4

8 medium carrots, sliced
1 tablespoon maple syrup

Steam carrots until soft. Top with maple syrup and serve. Carrots are an excellent source of beta carotene, an important nutrient for cancer protection.

Green Beans and Almonds *Serves 4*

1 pound green beans
2 ounces raw almonds, chopped
2 tablespoons flax oil
1/4 teaspoon sea salt

Steam green beans until tender. Toss with the almond bits, flax oil and sea salt for a buttery flavor. If you don't care for the taste of flax oil, a vinaigrette may be substituted. Flax oil may also be used to dress a variety of other vegetables.

Rice and Tofu Tabouli *Serves 6*

2 cups cooked brown rice
1 cup parsley, chopped
1/2 cup fresh mint, chopped
1/2 medium red onion, diced
1 medium tomato, diced
2 ounces firm tofu, diced
1 lemon, juiced
2 tablespoons olive oil
1/4 teaspoon sea salt
1 teaspoon cumin
1 teaspoon oregano

Place rice in a bowl. Mix in parsley, mint, red onion, tomato and diced tofu. Combine these ingredient well. Add lemon juice and olive oil and mix. Add cumin, oregano and salt to the salad and mix well. This is the ultimate delicious and healthy tabouli recipe. It is great served with the hummus and tahini recipe described below.

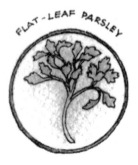

FLAT-LEAF PARSLEY

Hummus and Tahini

3/4 cup raw unhulled
    sesame seeds
1 cup water or cooking liquid
    from beans
1-3/4 cup garbanzo beans,
    cooked
1 clove of raw garlic
1 lemon, juiced
1/4 teaspoon salt

Grind sesame seeds into a powder using a seed or coffee grinder. Place to one side in a dish. Raw sesame butter available from most health food stores may be substituted. Combine water, garbanzo beans, ground sesame seeds, lemon juice, olive oil, garlic and salt in a food processor. Blend to the consistency of a smooth dip. Serve as a dip with pita bread, rye bread and fresh vegetables. This dip is an excellent source of essential fatty acids, calcium and easy-to-digest vegetable protein.

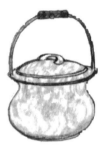

6 ounces black beans, cooked
6 ounces lentils or great
    northern beans, cooked
1/4 red pepper, diced
1/4 small red onion, diced
2 ounces celery, diced
1 cup brown rice
6 leaves romaine lettuce
2 tablespoons chopped green
    onions

Two-Bean Dish   *Serves 2*

In two separate bowls, combine each bean portion with half the red pepper, red onion and celery. Mix well. On a serving dish arrange leaves of romaine lettuce. Place the cup of brown rice in the center and arrange beans on either side. Sprinkle with chopped green onions and dress with oil and vinegar or your favorite vinaigrette dressing. Beans are an excellent source of calcium as well as easy-to-digest vegetable protein.

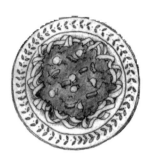

Pasta with Flax Oil and Garlic

Serves 4

1 pound pasta
1 clove garlic, minced
4 tablespoons flax oil
1 tablespoon soy Parmesan
   cheese (available at health
   food stores)
1 teaspoon basil
1/2 teaspoon sea salt

Cook pasta until tender. Top with garlic, flax oil, basil, salt and soy Parmesan. Mix until well blended and serve.

Tofu and Almond Stir Fry

Serves 4

3/4 cups firm tofu, cubed
1 cup raw almonds, chopped
1/2 red pepper, chopped
1/4 yellow onion, chopped
1/4 cup water
1 teaspoon sesame or
   safflower oil
3 cups brown rice, cooked
1 teaspoon wheat-free
   (tamari) soy sauce

Combine tofu, almonds, onions and red peppers in a large frying pan with water and oil. Cook over low flame for 5 minutes. (Add extra water to pan if needed.) Add rice to pan and mix. Heat for 5 minutes or until warm. Transfer to serving dish and toss with wheat-free soy sauce.

4 corn tortillas

3/4 pound pinto beans,
    cooked and pureed

1/4 pound soft tofu, mashed

1/2 avocado, thinly sliced

1/4 red onion, finely chopped

1/4 sweet red pepper, diced

1 tomato, diced

6 tablespoons salsa

1/2 head red or romaine
    lettuce, chopped

Vegetarian Tacos *Serves 4*

Warm tortillas and beans in separate pans. Place tortillas on individual serving dishes and spread with beans and tofu. Garnish with avocado, pepper, tomato and onion, then cover each taco with lettuce and 1-1/2 tablespoons of salsa.

4 fillets of salmon, 3 ounces
    each

1 cup water

1 lemon

Poached Salmon *Serves 4*

Combine water and juice of one lemon in skillet and heat. Place the salmon in the hot liquid. Cover and poach for 6 to 8 minutes or until the salmon flakes easily with a fork. Remove the fish and keep it warm until ready to serve.

2 fresh trout fillets, 6–8 ounces
    each

2 tablespoons lemon juice

chopped fresh dill (dried if
    fresh is unavailable)

Broiled Trout *Serves 4*

Slice each fillet in half. This will make four servings of trout. Sprinkle the fillets with lemon juice and dill. Place the trout in a broiler pan. Broil for 5 to 6 minutes or until done.

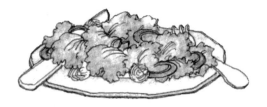

Substitute Healthy Ingredients in Recipes

Many recipes you have now probably contain ingredients that women with menopausal symptoms should avoid, such as caffeine, alcohol, sugar, chocolate and dairy products. Learning how to make substitutions for high-stress ingredients in familiar recipes allows you to make your favorite foods without compromising your emotional or physical health.

Some women choose to totally eliminate high-stress ingredients from a recipe. For example, you can make a pasta with tomato sauce but eliminate the Parmesan cheese topping and use nonwheat pasta. Greek salad can be made without the feta cheese. You may even make pizza without cheese, layering tomato sauce and lots of vegetables on the crust. In many cases, the high-stress ingredients are not necessary to make foods taste good; always remember, they can make your anxiety symptoms worse and impair your health.

If you want to use a particular high-stress ingredient, you can usually substantially reduce the amount of that ingredient you use, while still retaining the flavor and taste. Most of us have palates jaded by too much fat, salt, sugar and other flavorings. In many dishes, we taste only the additives; we never really enjoy the delicious flavors of the foods themselves. Now that I regularly substitute low-stress ingredients in my cooking, I enjoy the subtle taste of the dishes much more, and my health and vitality continue to improve. The following information tells you how to easily substitute healthy ingredients in your own recipes.

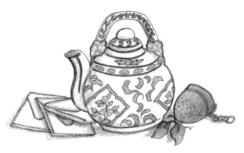

Caffeinated Foods and Beverages

Drink substitutes for coffee and black tea. The best substitutes are the grain-based coffee beverages, such as Pero, Postum and Cafix. Some women may find the abrupt discontinuance of coffee difficult because of withdrawal symptoms, such as headaches. If this concerns you, decrease your total coffee intake gradually to one or one-half cup per day. Use coffee substitutes for your other cups. This will help prevent withdrawal symptoms.

Use decaffeinated coffee or tea as a transition beverage. If you cannot give up coffee, start by substituting water-processed decaffeinated coffee for the real thing. Then try to wean yourself from coffee altogether or go to a coffee substitute.

Use herbal teas for energy and vitality. Many women with anxiety and excessive stress that may accompany menopause mistakenly drink coffee as a pick-me-up to be able to function during the day. Use ginger instead. It is a great herbal stimulant that won't damage your health. To make ginger tea, grate a few teaspoons of fresh ginger root into a pot of hot water; boil and steep. Serve with honey.

Substitute carob for chocolate. Unsweetened carob tastes like chocolate but doesn't contain the anxiety-causing caffeine found in chocolate. A member of the legume family, carob is high in calcium. You can purchase it in chunk form as a substitute for chocolate candy or as a powder for use in baking or drinks. Be careful, however, not to overindulge; carob, like chocolate, is high in calories and fat. Consider it a treat and an excellent cooking aid for use in small amounts only.

Sugar

Substitute concentrated sweeteners. Americans use too much sugar, which only increases symptoms of nervous tension, a problem during early menopause. I have found that as women decrease their sugar intake, most begin to enjoy the subtle flavors of the foods they eat. Concentrated sweeteners such as honey and maple syrup have a sweeter taste per quantity used than table sugar. Using these substitutes will allow you to decrease the amount of table sugar you use in a recipe. If you use a concentrated sweetener in place of sugar in the average recipe, reduce the liquid content in the recipe by one-fourth cup. If no liquid is used in the recipe, add three to five tablespoons of flour for each three-fourths cup of concentrated sweetener.

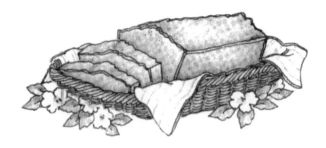

Substitute fruit for sugar in baked goods. When making muffins and cookies, you may want to try deleting sugar altogether and adding extra fruits and nuts.

Alcohol

Use low-alcohol or nonalcoholic products for drinking or cooking. There are many low- and nonalcoholic wines and beers available in supermarkets and liquor stores. Many of these taste quite good and can be used for meals or other social occasions. In addition, you can substitute low-alcohol or nonalcoholic wine or beer when cooking or preparing sauces and marinades. You will retain much of the flavor that alcohol imparts, and you'll decrease the stress factor substantially.

Dairy Products

Eliminate or decrease the amount of cow's milk cheese you use in food preparation and cooking. If you must use cow's milk cheese in cooking, decrease the amount in the recipe by three-fourths so that it becomes a flavoring or garnish rather than a major source of fat and protein. For example, use one teaspoon of Parmesan cheese on top of a casserole instead of one-half cup.

Use soy cheese in food preparation and cooking. Soy cheese is an excellent substitute for cow's milk cheese. It is lower in fat and salt, and the fat it does contain isn't saturated. Women with severe fatigue may have difficulty digesting it, so I recommend its use only to women who do not suffer from severe fatigue. Health food stores offer many brands and flavors, such as mozzarella, cheddar, American and jack. The quality of these products keeps improving all the time. You can use soy cheese as a perfect cheese substitute in sandwiches, salads, pizzas, lasagnas and casseroles. In some recipes you can replace cheese with soft tofu. I have done this often with lasagna, layering the lasagna noodles with tofu and topping with melted soy cheese for a delicious dish.

Replace milk and yogurt in recipes. For cow's milk, substitute potato milk, soy milk, nut milk or grain milk. One of my personal favorites is Vegelicious,® a nondairy milk made from an all-vegetable potato base. It is creamy and sweet and tastes very similar to the best cow's milk, with none of the unhealthy characteristics of dairy products. Even my 11-year-old daughter likes it. The potato-based milk is high in calcium and can be bought either in liquid or powder form.. It stores well and mixes easily in water; it can be used exactly as you use cow's milk for beverages, cooking and baking. Soy milk and nut milk are available at most health food stores. Many nondairy milks are good sources of calcium and can be used for drinking, eating or baking.

For cow's milk-based yogurt, substitute soy yogurt. Several excellent brands of soy yogurt are available in health food stores in plain, vanilla and various fruit flavors. Its great taste approximates cow's milk yogurt. Soy yogurt works well for both cooking and baking.

Substitute flax oil for butter. Flax oil is the best substitute for butter I've found: a rich, golden oil that looks and tastes like butter. It is delicious on anything you'd normally top with butter—toast, rice, popcorn, steamed vegetables or potatoes. Flax oil is extremely high in essential fatty acids—the type of fat that is very healthy for a woman's body. Essential fatty acids improve vitality, enhance circulation, and help promote normal hormonal function. Flax oil is very perishable, however, because it is sensitive to heat and light. You can't cook with it—cook the food first and add the flax oil before serving. Also, keep it refrigerated. Flax oil has so many health benefits that I highly recommend its use; it can be found in health food stores.

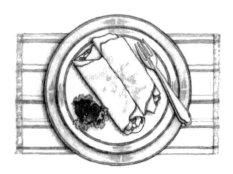

Red Meat and Poultry

Substitute beans, tofu or seeds in recipes. You can often modify recipes calling for hamburger or ground turkey by substituting tofu. For example, crumble up the tofu to simulate the texture of hamburger and add to recipes for enchiladas, tacos, chili and ground beef casseroles. The tofu absorbs the flavor of the sauce used in the dish and is indistinguishable from meat. Tofu can even be frozen (ideally for one to two weeks) to improve its texture as a meat substitute. Once defrosted, tofu will crumble like hamburger when used in appropriate recipes. In addition, many substitute meat products are available in natural food stores. These products include tofu hot dogs, hamburger, bacon, ham, chicken and turkey. The variety is astounding and many of these imitation meat products taste remarkably good. Also, the quality of these products has dramatically improved in the past few years.

When making salads that call for meat, such as chef's salad or Cobb salad, substitute kidney beans, garbanzo beans and sunflower seeds. These provide the needed protein, yet are more easily digested than meats. You can also sprinkle sunflower seeds on top of casseroles for extra protein and essential fatty acids. When making stir-fries, substitute tofu, almonds or sprouts for beef or chicken. Vegetable protein-based stir-fries taste delicious!

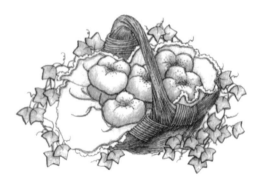

Wheat Flour

Use whole grain, nonwheat flour. Substitute whole grain, nonwheat flours, such as rice or barley flour. Whole grain flours are much higher in essential nutrients, such as vitamin B complex and many minerals. They are also higher in fiber content. Rice flour makes excellent cookies, cakes and other pastries. Barley flour is the best for pie crusts.

Salt

Substitute potassium-based products for table salt (sodium chloride). Potassium-based products, such as Morton's Salt Substitute, are much healthier and will not aggravate heart disease or hypertension.

Use powdered seaweed such as kelp or nori to season vegetables, grains and salads. They are high in essential iodine and trace elements.

Use herbs instead of salt for flavoring. Herbs have subtle flavors that will help even the most jaded palate appreciate the taste of fresh fruits, vegetables and meats.

Use liquid flavoring agents with advertised low-sodium content. Low-salt soy sauce and Bragg's Amino Acids, a liquid soybean-based flavoring agent, are delicious when used as salt substitutes in cooking. Add them to soups, casseroles, stir-fries and other dishes at the end of the cooking process. You need only a small amount for intense flavoring.

Substitutes for Common High-Stress Ingredients

High-Stress Ingredient	Low-Stress Substitute
3/4 cup sugar	1/2 cup honey
	1/4 cup molasses
	1/2 cup maple syrup
	1/2 oz. barley malt
	1 cup apple butter
	2 cups apple juice
1 cup milk	1 cup soy, potato, nut, or grain milk
1 cup yogurt	1 cup soy yogurt
1 tablespoon butter	1 tablespoon flax oil (must be used raw and unheated)
1/2 teaspoon salt	1 tablespoon miso
	1/2 teaspoon potassium chloride salt substitute
	1/2 teaspoon Mrs. Dash, Spike
	1/2 teaspoon herbs (basil, tarragon, oregano, etc.)
1-1/2 cups cocoa	1 cup powdered carob
1 square chocolate	3/4 tablespoon powdered carob
1 tablespoon coffee	1 tablespoon decaffeinated coffee
	1 tablespoon Pero, Postum, Caffix, or other grain-based coffee substitute
4 oz. wine	4 oz. light wine
8 oz. beer	8 oz. near beer
1 cup wheat flour	1 cup barley flour (pie crust)
	1 cup rice flour (cookies, cakes, breads)
1 cup meat	1 cup beans, tofu
	1/4 cup seeds

12

Vitamins, Minerals & Essential Fatty Acids

$\mathcal{N}$utritional supplements can provide an effective alternative to estrogen for many menopausal women who cannot or do not choose to use prescription hormones. In addition, nutritional supplements when used as part of a complete life-style-based program (in combination with medication or hormonal therapy when appropriate), will help reduce the incidence and prevent the onset of many common problems seen after midlife such as heart disease and loss of bone mass.

The important role nutritional supplements can play in helping reduce the symptoms of premenopause and menopause as well as the risk of common postmenopausal health problems is supported by many medical research studies done at university centers and hospitals (a bibliography is provided at the end of this book).

The use of supplements must go hand-in-hand with a low-stress, healthful diet. It is not enough to take supplements while continuing poor dietary habits. Women who try this do not achieve the results they're looking for. However, diet alone often cannot provide the nutrient levels necessary for the most complete relief of menopausal symptoms. Supplements can speed up and facilitate the return to optimal health and well-being.

This chapter is divided into two sections. In the first section, the role of vitamins, minerals and essential fatty acids in symptom relief and prevention is discussed. In the second section, I provide specific recommendations, usage tips, and optimal nutritional formulas for premenopausal and menopausal women. Also included are charts listing major food sources of each essential nutrient discussed.

Vitamins and Minerals for Relieving Menopausal Symptoms

In this section, I give specific information about vitamins, minerals and essential fatty acids that are most useful for the relief and prevention of specific menopause-related problems.

Heavy and Irregular Bleeding

Vitamin A. Heavy menstrual bleeding is a significant problem for premenopausal women due to the production of excessive amounts of estrogen or the accelerated growth of fibroids. Excessive bleeding is also one of the most common reasons for hysterectomies. Luckily, vitamin A can play a role in reducing these symptoms.

In a study of 71 women with excessive bleeding, the women had significantly lower blood levels of vitamin A than the average population. After two weeks of vitamin A treatment, almost 90 percent of the women studied returned to a normal bleeding pattern. Vitamin A promotes normal growth and support for the eyes, skin, mucous membranes, red blood cells and healthy immune function. Deficiency of vitamin A results in impaired immune function, rough, scaly skin and night blindness.

Vitamin A is found in two forms. Vitamin A from animal sources, usually from fish liver, is oil soluble. This type of vitamin A can be toxic if taken in too large a dose (greater than 25,000 international units [IU] per day for more than a few months). In contrast, beta carotene, the precursor of vitamin A found in plants, is water soluble and is not toxic in large amounts. A single sweet potato or cup of carrot juice contains more than 20,000 IU of beta carotene.

Vitamin B Complex. Vitamin B complex consists of 11 factors that perform many important biochemical functions in the body. These include stabilization of brain chemistry, glucose metabolism and the inactivation of estrogen by the liver. Since heavy menstrual bleeding can be triggered by excess estrogen in the body, it is important that estrogen levels are properly regulated through breakdown and disposal by the liver. In pioneering animal and human research in 1942 and 1943, M. S. Biskind highlighted the important role of several B-complex vitamins in regulating estrogen levels through promoting healthy liver function. Women with several problems related to excessive estrogen levels, including heavy menstrual flow, PMS and fibrocystic breast disease received supplements of vitamin B complex. When supplemented with thiamine (B_1), riboflavin (B_2), niacin and niacinamide (B_3), as well as the rest of the B complex, the women in this research study showed relief from estrogen-related symptoms.

In women with heavy menstrual bleeding, I generally recommend 50 to 100 mg per day of vitamin B complex. The B vitamins are water soluble and easily lost from the body. Emotional and nutritional stress accelerate the loss of these essential nutrients from the body. This can increase other symptoms seen with fibroids and endometriosis including fatigue, faintness and dizziness. Besides supplementation, a diet high in B complex is desirable for women. The B-complex vitamins are commonly found in food such as whole grains, beans, peas and liver.

Vitamin C. Vitamin C has been tested, along with bioflavonoids, as a treatment for heavy menstrual bleeding. One research project showed a reduction in bleeding in 87 percent of the women participating in the study. Dozens of similar studies showing the efficacy of vitamin C and bioflavonoids for the treatment of heavy bleeding. Vitamin C reduces bleeding by strengthening capillaries. Women who bleed excessively may eventually become iron deficient and develop anemia. Vitamin C increases iron absorption from food sources such as bran, peas, seeds, nuts and leafy green vegetables, thus helping prevent iron-deficiency anemia. I recommend that women with excessive bleeding use 1000 to 4000 mg of vitamin C per day, especially when symptoms occur. Many fruits and vegetables are excellent sources of vitamin C.

Bioflavonoids. Like vitamin C, bioflavonoids (also called vitamin P) have shown dramatic ability to reduce heavy menstrual bleeding through strengthening the capillary walls. Bioflavonoids have the additional property of being weakly estrogenic and anti-estrogenic, important properties for control of heavy bleeding due to elevated estrogen levels. Bioflavonoids contain estrogen but at doses much weaker than in drugs. The bioflavonoids help to normalize estrogen levels, reducing them in women who suffer from excessive levels, and boosting them in women who are deficient.

I generally recommend 500 to 2000 mg bioflavonoids per day in women with premenopausal bleeding problems. On one hand, bioflavonoids compete for space on the binding sites of enzymes needed for estrogen production with the estrogen precursors produced by your body. In this way they lower estrogen levels in women with heavy menstrual bleeding. On the other hand, the weakly estrogenic effect of the bioflavonoids can help relieve symptoms such as hot flashes, night sweats and mood swings in menopausal women who are grossly deficient in estrogen. Bioflavonoids are found in grape skins, cherries, blackberries and blueberries as well as being abundant in citrus fruits, especially in the pulp and the white rind. They are also found in other foods such as buckwheat and soybeans.

Iron. Women who suffer from premenopausal heavy menstrual bleeding run the risk of developing iron deficiency, the main cause of anemia. Iron is an essential component of red blood cells, combining with protein and copper to make hemoglobin, the pigment of the red blood cells. Iron deficiency is common during all phases of a woman's life and is a frequent cause of fatigue and low-energy states. In fact, some medical studies have found that inadequate iron intake may cause excessive bleeding.

Women who suffer from heavy menstrual bleeding should have their red blood count checked to see if supplemental iron is necessary, in addition to a high-iron-content diet. Heme iron, the iron from meat sources such as liver, is much better absorbed and assimilated than nonheme iron, the iron from vegetarian sources. To be absorbed properly, nonheme iron must be taken with at least 75 mg of vitamin C.

Good food sources of iron include liver, blackstrap molasses, beans, peas, seeds, nuts, certain fruits and vegetables.

Hot Flashes, Night Sweats, Vaginal and Bladder Atrophy

Vitamin A. Vitamin A is necessary for the growth and support of the skin and mucous membranes. As a result, this nutrient is very important for the support of the vulvar, vaginal and urinary tissues. Lack of vitamin A is a risk factor for developing bladder or cervical cancer and can predispose a woman to skin conditions related to the aging process, such as vulvar leukoplakia and senile keratosis. Both of these conditions can precede the onset of skin cancer.

Vitamin A is best from the vegetable source, beta carotene. This is because vitamin A from animal sources can produce toxic symptoms such as headaches and liver damage if taken in excessive doses for periods longer than several months. However, the provitamin A, beta carotene, is extremely safe. For women with vaginal and bladder atrophy, I generally recommend between 25,000 to 100,000 IU per day. (25,000 IU is found in one sweet potato or one cup of carrot juice.)

Vitamin C. Adequate amounts of vitamin C are needed to maintain the skin, including the vulvar, vaginal and bladder tissues. Vitamin C is necessary for collagen synthesis and skin strength. A low vitamin C intake has been found to predispose women to cervical dysplasia and cancer of the cervix.

The diet of women with early-stage cervical cancer has been compared to those of healthy controls in medical research studies. The women with cervical cancer were found to have a diet much lower in foods containing vitamin C. While vitamin C alone will not reverse bladder and vaginal atrophy, sufficient daily intake of this nutrient is necessary, along with vitamin A, for the continued support of these tissues.

I generally recommend between 1000 to 5000 mg per day for menopausal women. Side effects are rare, although some women find that higher doses cause diarrhea; if this happens to you, reduce the dose to a comfortable level. Rarely, large doses of vitamin C can predispose to kidney stones. If you have a history of kidney stones, keep your vitamin C intake well below 5000 mg per day and drink lots of water. If you have any questions about these issues, ask your physician. Many women use vitamin C, even at high doses, with no side effects and derive many health benefits from its use. Vitamin C is found abundantly in nature in a variety of foods. Many fruits and vegetables as well as some meats contain high levels of vitamin C.

Bioflavonoids. While bioflavonoids can be very useful in helping relieve and prevent premenopausal symptoms, they can be equally useful for menopausal women. This is because bioflavonoids are weakly estrogenic and can be used as a safe, nontoxic substitute for estrogen. As mentioned earlier, the potencies of bioflavonoids are so low (1/50,000 that of stilbestrol, a synthetic estrogen), that they have no side effects for most women, yet can help relieve hot flashes as well as vaginal dryness. One study of 94 women at Loyola University Medical School showed the effectiveness of a bioflavonoids-vitamin C combination in controlling hot flashes for most of the women tested. In addition, bioflavonoids were suggested in this particular study as an estrogen substitute for cancer patients who cannot use traditional replacement therapy because their tumors are estrogen-sensitive. The low rate of breast cancer among Japanese women, whose soy-based diet is high in bioflavonoids, is thought to be a testimony to the benefits of this nutrient. As mentioned in the chapter on diet, when a nutritional program based on soy and flax seeds was used for women with vaginal atrophy, this regimen helped build up and thicken the vaginal lining. Women who don't wish to eat a soy-based diet but would like relief from vaginal and hot flash symptoms can use bioflavonoids in a purified form as a nutritional supplement. The usual dose varies from 500 to 2000 mg.

Vitamin E. Vitamin E has shown promise in research studies as a treatment for the most common menopausal symptoms, including hot flashes, night sweats and even vaginal dryness. Depending on the study, between 66 to 80 percent of the women tested found vitamin E to be an effective substitute for estrogen. Vitamin E can be a useful treatment option for women who cannot or do not choose to use the higher potencies of prescription hormones. For example, one early research study in *The American Journal of Obstetrics and Gynecology* reported that nearly all 25 cancer patients they studied had an excellent response to vitamin E therapy. These women had become menopausal either through surgery or reduced dosage of hormone replacement. All had severe hot flashes and mood alterations that could not be treated by estrogen replacement therapy due to their types of tumors. Using vitamin E as an estrogen substitute, 23 out of the 25 women had either complete relief or significant improvement of their symptoms.

Another interesting study of 47 menopausal women reported in the *British Medical Journal* found that vitamin E not only helped reduce hot flashes in 64 percent of women tested, but also helped reduce symptoms of vaginal aging. Fifty percent of the women noted healing of vaginal atrophy as well as a decrease in pain during sexual intercourse. To repeat for emphasis, many women with vaginal atrophy are also prone to recurrent vaginal infections which produce uncomfortable symptoms such as itching, burning and discharge. A study in *The American Journal of Obstetrics and Gynecology* reported that 44 women at high risk for developing yeast vaginitis because of a pre-existing diabetic condition noted significant relief of symptoms when treated with vitamin E vaginal suppositories.

Generally, I recommend using 400 to 2400 IU of vitamin E per day. Begin at a low dose and gradually increase the dosage over several weeks until you achieve the desired relief. Women with hypertension, diabetes or bleeding problems, however, should begin at much lower dosages of vitamin E (100 IU per day). If you have any of these conditions, ask your physician about the advisability of using vitamin E. In general, however, vitamin E tends to be well tolerated and is used by millions of people without adverse effects. Many women with severe vaginal atrophy use vitamin E topically. Besides taking vitamin E by mouth, you might try opening a capsule and applying the oil directly to your vaginal tissues. Vitamin E occurs abundantly in vegetable oils, raw nuts, seeds and in some fruits and vegetables.

Essential Fatty Acids. Essential fatty acids are particularly important to menopausal women because the deficiency of these oils is responsible, in part, for the drying of the vaginal and bladder mucosa as well as the skin, hair and other tissues of the body that occur at midlife. The deficiency is primarily nutritional because these fats cannot be made by the body and must be supplied daily in your diet. The main sources of essential fatty acids are raw seeds and nuts or fish, which are not a usual part of the typical American (or Western) diet.

Both whole ground flax seeds, which are 50 percent oil by content, or purified oil in capsule form are excellent sources of the two essential oils linoleic acid and linolenic acid. Flax meal was the oil source used in the study of vaginal atrophy reported in the *British Medical Journal* in 1990, though many women prefer to take essential fatty acids in capsule form. Other excellent sources of essential fatty acids include evening primrose oil, borage oil and black currant oil. Unlike flax oil, these other oils are not used as food, but as nutritional supplements. I find that two to eight capsules per day, at least in the early stages, work best when trying to replace moisture and softness in the skin. Alternatively, women who like the buttery taste of raw flax oil may want to take one to three tablespoons orally per day of flax oil.

Menopause-Related Emotional Symptoms and Insomnia

Vitamin B complex. The B vitamins play an important role in healthy nervous system function. When one or more of these vitamins are deficient, symptoms of nerve impairment, anxiety, stress and fatigue can result. Conversely, eating appropriate food sources and taking supplements of B vitamins can help calm the mood and provide important factors for a stable and constant source of energy. This can be very important during menopause when women's moods tend to fluctuate due to hormonal instability.

Consistent high levels of emotional stress trigger the fight-or-flight alarm response which results in excessive output of adrenal hormones. Deficiencies of individual B vitamins also increase nervous tension and stress. Pantothenic acid (vitamin B_5) is needed for healthy adrenal function. Pyridoxine (vitamin B_6) also affects mood because it has an important role in the conversion of linoleic acid to gamma linolenic acid (GLA) in the production of the beneficial series-one prostaglandins. Prostaglandins have a relaxant effect on both mood and smooth muscle tissue. Lack of these relaxant hormones has been linked to stress-related problems such as irritable bowel syndrome and migraine headaches.

Vitamin B_6 levels may decrease in menopausal women who are using estrogen replacement therapy. (This can also be a problem for women using oral contraceptives, a common treatment for PMS, menstrual cramps and irregularity.) Anxiety symptoms can occur as a side effect of hormone use in both groups of women, in part because of B_6 deficiency. Vitamin B_6 can be safely used in doses up to 300 mg; doses above this level can be neurotoxic and should be avoided or used under a physician's care.

Lack of B_6 may also increase anxiety symptoms directly through its effect on the nervous system. The body needs B_6 in order to convert the amino acid tryptophan to serotonin, an important neurotransmitter. Serotonin regulates sleep; when it is deficient, insomnia occurs. Sleeplessness is a condition menopausal women frequently suffer. Serotonin levels also strongly affect mood and social behavior. Both B_6 and food sources of tryptophan such as almonds, pumpkin seeds, sesame seeds and certain other protein-containing foods, are necessary for adequate serotonin production.

For women who fall asleep easily but can't return to sleep after awakening in the middle of the night, niacin (vitamin B_3) may be helpful. Research studies have shown that niacinamide, a form of niacin, has effects similar to those in minor tranquilizers. In addition, inositol, another B vitamin, has been shown to have calming effects. Its effect on brain waves studied by electroencephalograph (EEG) were similar to changes induced by minor tranquilizers.

In summary, the entire range of B vitamins is needed in order to provide nutritional support to avoid anxiety and stress symptoms. Because B vitamins are water soluble, the body cannot readily store them. Thus, B vitamins must be consumed daily through diet. Good sources of most B vitamins include brewer's yeast (which many women cannot easily digest), liver, whole grain germ and bran, beans, peas and nuts. Vitamin B_{12} is found primarily in animal foods. Women following a vegan diet (a vegetarian diet utilizing no dairy products or eggs) should take particular care to add supplemental vitamin B_{12} to their diets.

Vitamin C. Vitamin C is an extremely important antistress nutrient that can help decrease the fatigue symptoms that often accompany excessive levels of nervous tension and stress. It is needed for the production of adrenal gland hormones. Activation of the fight-or-flight pattern in response to stress depletes these hormones. Larger amounts of vitamin C in the diet are needed when stress levels are high. In one research study done on 411 dentists and their spouses, scientists found a clear relationship between lack of vitamin C and the presence of fatigue.

The best sources of vitamin C in nature are fruits and vegetables. It is a water-soluble vitamin, so it is not stored in the body. Thus, menopausal women with anxiety and excessive stress should replenish their vitamin C supply daily through a healthy diet and the use of supplements.

Bioflavonoids. As mentioned earlier, bioflavonoids have the property of being weakly estrogenic, which is helpful for the stress due to menopause-related hormonal deficiency. Since estrogen has a stimulant effect on the brain, the weakly estrogenic activity of the bioflavonoids can act as a mild mood elevator in hormonally deficient women. In nature, bioflavonoids can be found along with vitamin C in fruits and vegetables. (See the preceding sections for food sources as well as preferred dosages of this helpful nutrient.)

Vitamin E. Like bioflavonoids, vitamin E relieves symptoms of anxiety and mood swings triggered by an estrogen-progesterone imbalance. This can occur in women suffering from either menopause or PMS. In studies of vitamin E as an alternative treatment for menopause, it has relieved mood swings and reduced other menopause-related symptoms. In one interesting study on 66 women with menopause-related psychological symptoms including depression, tearfulness and irritability, as well as hot flashes, 60 women had a significant therapeutic response to vitamin E, with relief of their emotional symptoms. Some women find that conventional estrogen therapy increases their anxiety symptoms because the available medication doses do not match their physical needs. These women are potentially good candidates for vitamin E therapy.

The best natural sources of vitamin E are wheat germ oil, walnut oil and soy bean oil. I generally recommend that women with menopause-related anxiety and mood swings use between 400 to 2000 IU per day. Women with hypertension, diabetes, or bleeding problems should start on a much lower dose of vitamin E (100 IU per day); if you have any of these conditions, ask your physician about the advisability of these supplements. Any increase in dosage should be made slowly and monitored carefully in these women. Otherwise, vitamin E tends to be extremely safe and is commonly used.

Magnesium. The body requires adequate levels of magnesium in order to maintain energy and vitality. In menopausal women, magnesium is required in order to produce ATP (adenosine triphosphate), the end product of the conversion of food to usable energy by the body's cells. ATP is the universal energy currency the body uses to run hundreds of thousands of chemical reactions. The digestive system can extract this energy from food efficiently only in the presence of magnesium, oxygen and other nutrients. When magnesium is deficient, ATP production falls and the body forms lactic acid instead. Researchers have linked excessive accumulation of lactic acid with anxiety and irritability symptoms.

Magnesium also facilitates conversion of the essential fatty acid linoleic acid to gamma linolenic acid and its conversion to the beneficial relaxant prostaglandin hormones. These hormones help reduce anxiety and mood-swing symptoms in susceptible women.

Many menopausal women feel depressed and tired due to the chemical and hormonal changes occurring at this time. Medical research studies on the treatment of fatigue use a special form of magnesium called magnesium aspartate, formed by combining magnesium with aspartic acid. Aspartic acid also plays an important role in the production of energy in the body and helps transport magnesium and potassium into the cells. In a number of clinical studies, magnesium aspartate, along with potassium aspartate, has been shown to reduce fatigue after five to six weeks of constant use. Many of those in the study began to feel better after just ten days. This beneficial effect was seen in 90 percent of those tested, a very high success rate.

Magnesium supplements can also benefit women who have menopause-related insomnia. When taken before bedtime, magnesium helps calm the mood and induce restful sleep. Good food sources of magnesium include green leafy vegetables, beans, peas, raw nuts and seeds, tofu, avocados, raisins, dried figs, millet and other grains. Menopausal women need 400 to 750 mg per day of magnesium, either from food sources or nutritional supplements, for their daily allowance.

Potassium. Like magnesium, potassium has a powerful enhancing effect on energy and vitality. Potassium deficiency has been associated with fatigue and muscular weakness. One study showed that older people deficient in potassium had weak grip strength. In a number of studies on chronic fatigue, potassium aspartate combined with magnesium aspartate significantly restored energy levels; this combination may be quite useful in menopausal women suffering from excessive fatigue and depression when mineral deficiencies coexist with the lack of hormones.

Potassium can be lost through chronic diarrhea or the overuse of diuretics. In addition, the excessive use of coffee and alcohol (both of which can magnify anxiety and emotional stress symptoms) increase the loss of potassium through the urinary tract.

For women suffering from potassium loss, the use of a potassium supplement may be helpful. The most common dose available is a 99 mg tablet or capsule. I generally recommend one to two per day during times of extreme stress and fatigue. Potassium, however, should be used cautiously. Women with kidney or cardiovascular disease should avoid potassium because high levels can cause an irregular heartbeat. Also, potassium can irritate the intestinal tract, so it should be taken with meals. If you have any questions about the proper use of this mineral, ask your health care provider. Potassium occurs in abundance in fruits, vegetables, beans and peas, seeds and nuts, starches and whole grains.

Calcium. Calcium is the most abundant mineral in the body. This important mineral helps combat stress, nervous tension and anxiety. An upset emotional state can dramatically increase tension and fatigue in susceptible women. A calcium deficiency increases not only emotional irritability but also muscular irritability and cramps. Calcium taken at night along with magnesium will reduce muscular cramps, calm the mood and induce a restful sleep in menopausal women. Women with menopause-related anxiety, mood swings and fatigue may find calcium supplements useful.

Many women consume less than the recommended daily allowance for calcium in their diet (800 mg for women during active reproductive years, 1200 to 1500 mg after menopause). In fact, many women only take in half the recommended amount through diet. In addition, anxiety and stress can inhibit calcium absorption, as will a high-fat diet, lack of exercise and other risk factors. As a result, a calcium supplement may be useful. Good food sources of calcium include green leafy vegetables, salmon (with bones), nuts, seeds, tofu and blackstrap molasses.

Zinc. Zinc is an essential trace mineral necessary for the absorption and assimilation of vitamins, especially the anxiety- and stress-combating B vitamins. It is a constituent of many enzymes involved in metabolism and digestion. Zinc helps reduce anxiety and upset in menopausal women when there is a coexisting blood sugar imbalance. This is due to zinc's role in normal carbohydrate digestion. Because diabetes becomes increasingly prevalent after menopause, support of carbohydrate metabolism is extremely important in midlife women. Zinc is a component of insulin, the protein that helps move glucose out of blood circulation and into the cells. Once inside the cells, glucose provides them with their main source of energy. Menopausal women may want to use between 15 and 25 mg of zinc per day in a supplemental form. Good food sources of zinc include soy meal, whole wheat, chicken, rice bran, black-eyed peas, buckwheat, cabbage, pumpkin seeds and peanut butter.

Chromium and Manganese. These two minerals are also important in carbohydrate production metabolism. Chromium helps keep the blood sugar level balanced by enhancing insulin function so that glucose is properly utilized by the body. This avoids the extremes of too little glucose in the blood (hypoglycemia) or too much glucose (diabetes mellitus). Improving the uptake of glucose into the cells allows these cells to use the glucose to produce energy. Manganese aids glucose metabolism by acting as a cofactor in the process of converting glucose (food) to energy.

Good sources of chromium include brewer's yeast (difficult for many women to digest), whole wheat, rye, oysters, potatoes, apples, bananas, spinach, molasses and chicken. Dietary sources of manganese are whole grains, nuts, beans, peas and green leafy vegetables. Many menopausal women (as well as men and women of all ages) lack adequate dietary sources of these nutrients. It is probably a good idea to use a high-potency multivitamin and mineral supplement in order to obtain sufficient amounts of these minerals on a daily basis.

Conditions Affected by Vitamins, Minerals and Essential Fatty Acids

Essential fatty acids are an extremely important part of the nutritional program for any women with menopause-related mood swings. Prostaglandins have muscle-relaxant and blood vessel-relaxant properties that will significantly reduce muscle cramps and tension. These can also be very useful for calming nervous tension in menopausal women. Essential fatty acids, because of their beneficial therapeutic effects on mood, have been used in the treatment of PMS, anxiety and eating disorders.

As mentioned earlier, there are two essential fatty acids, linoleic acid (Omega-6 family) and linolenic acid (Omega-3 family). They are derived from specific food sources in our diet, primarily raw seeds and nuts, and certain fish including salmon, mackerel and trout. Linoleic and linolenic acids are not made by the body and must be supplied daily in our diets, from either food or supplements. For women who wish to derive their fatty acid intake from nutritional supplements, many sources are readily available in natural food stores. These include encapsulated products such as evening primrose oil, borage oil, black currant oil and fish oil. Flax oil capsules contain both linoleic and linolenic acids so they are the most complete and well-balanced product. Otherwise, a mix of seed oil and fish oil capsules may be used in dosages ranging from one to six capsules per day, depending on need.

Osteoporosis

Calcium. Dozens of studies reinforce the importance of calcium for the prevention of osteoporosis. For example, a study completed in 1990 showed a group of premenopausal women whose spinal vertebrae bone loss averaged one percent a year. With increased intake of calcium-rich foods, further bone loss was prevented. Calcium is the most abundant mineral in the body, and 99 percent of it is deposited in the bones and teeth. (The other one percent is involved in blood clotting, nerve and muscle stimulation, and other important functions.) As a result, calcium is the most important structural mineral in bone. However, calcium absorption becomes much less efficient by the time women reach their postmenopausal years due to aging of the digestive tract. Calcium needs an acid environment in the stomach for proper digestion and, unfortunately, as many as 40 percent of postmenopausal women lack sufficient stomach acid for proper calcium absorption.

The average American woman takes in 400 to 500 mg per day. This is far less than the recommended daily allowance (RDA) of 800 mg per day for women during their active reproductive years and the 1200 to 1500 mg per day needed by postmenopausal women. Both the National Institutes of Health and the National Osteoporosis Foundation recommend that postmenopausal women take 1500 mg daily to compensate for calcium loss. To compound this problem, calcium absorption is inefficient and only 20 to 30 percent of the calcium ingested is utilized by the body.

As a result, adequate calcium supplementation as well as the specific type of calcium used is of major importance for most women. The main type of calcium supplements has been calcium carbonate. This is an alkaline form of calcium and is not absorbed well. In contrast, calcium citrate, an acidified form of calcium, is well-absorbed and a good source of the nutrient for women wishing to prevent bone loss. Be sure to check the label of any calcium supplement to make sure the dosages and the type of calcium used are optimal for your needs.

Phosphorus. Phosphorus is the second most abundant mineral in the body, found in bones and soft tissues. A major structural mineral of bone, it is present in the bones in a specific ratio of 2.5 parts calcium to 1 part phosphorus. This balance is important for both minerals to be used efficiently by the body. Because the American diet contains abundant phosphorus in foods such as meat, eggs, grains, seeds, nuts and soft drinks, phosphorus deficiency is relatively rare. In addition, phosphorus is easily absorbed from the digestive tract with an approximately 70 percent absorption rate. The RDA for phosphorus is 800 mg.

Magnesium. While not as prevalent as either calcium or phosphorus in bone, magnesium is equally important for healthy bones. Mild magnesium deficiency may be a risk factor in the development of osteoporosis. Magnesium is needed for bone growth as well as proper calcium absorption and assimilation. If the body does not have enough magnesium available, it deposits calcium pathologically in tissues and organs, so calcium accumulates in the muscles, heart and kidneys. In susceptible women, calcium deposited in the kidneys can cause kidney stones. As a result, a woman increasing her calcium intake should also increase magnesium intake in a ratio of either 2:1 or 10:4 calcium to magnesium. Other minerals, such as zinc, copper, manganese and silicon, are also needed in trace amounts for healthy bone growth and regulation of bone metabolism.

Vitamin D. Vitamin D is a fat soluble vitamin that can either be ingested in the diet or formed on the skin through exposure to sunlight. Sunlight activates a type of cholesterol found in the skin, converting it to vitamin D.

Vitamin D helps prevent osteoporosis by aiding in the absorption of calcium from the intestinal tract. It is needed for the synthesis of enzymes found in mucous membranes which are used in the active transport of calcium. A secondary advantage of taking the proper amounts of calcium and vitamin D, noted in a study of 35,216 women, is that these two nutrients have been shown to have a preventative effect on colon cancer, second to lung cancer as a cause of death in the United States.

Vitamin D also helps break down and assimilate phosphorus. A deficiency of vitamin D causes inadequate absorption of calcium from the intestinal tract as well as retention of phosphorus by the kidneys. This causes an imbalance in the calcium-phosphorus ratio, leading to faulty mineralization of the bones. Vitamin D is usually included in multivitamin products and is also found in fish liver oil supplements (along with vitamin A) and fortified milk. Menopausal women should have 400 IU per day of vitamin D.

Cardiovascular Disease

Beta Carotene. Oxygen-related damage to LDL cholesterol has been linked to the development of cardiovascular disease. Laboratory and clinical studies suggest that beta carotene can prevent this oxygen-related damage and thereby help protect the blood vessels from the disease process. Beta carotene does this by inactivating singlet oxygen, a free radical and a form of oxygen that is unstable. When these unstable free radicals attack cells in the body (including the circulatory system) to gain a second electron, they can damage chromosomes, alter the collagen process and accelerate the aging process. While the protective benefits of beta carotene, a so-called antioxidant, have not been definitely proven, the studies to date suggest that the use of beta carotene may be beneficial. The U.S. Physicians' Health Study found in a group of 333 participants with chest pain but no prior history of heart attack that beta carotene appeared to have a protective effect. Fifty percent fewer major cardiovascular events occurred, including heart attacks, strokes and cardiac related deaths. I recommend the use of beta carotene or beta carotene-containing foods because of its many benefits for good health, aside from any possible cardiovascular protection.

Vitamin C. Like beta carotene, vitamin C is a water-soluble vitamin that appears to be helpful in preventing LDL cholesterol oxidation, a process that can initiate atherogenesis (the destruction of the blood vessel wall and the formation of plaque) and eventually cause major incidents such as heart attacks and strokes. In the Nurses Health Study, in which over 87,000 women between the ages of 34 and 54 were studied, the association between dietary intake of vitamin C and the risk of developing coronary artery disease was evaluated. The risk of developing heart disease was more than 42 percent lower for women who used high doses of vitamin C than for women with a low vitamin C intake. Another study in Boston found that both males and females using vitamin C supplementation had lower levels of blood pressure, lower LDL cholesterol and higher HDL cholesterol (the type of cholesterol that confers protection against coronary artery disease) than participants with a lower vitamin C intake. Vitamin C is also necessary for the regeneration of vitamin E in the body, another important antioxidant nutrient. These results make a good case for vitamin C cardiovascular protective effects.

A dose between 1000 and 5000 mg of vitamin C can be quite useful for its protective effects on the body. Good food sources of vitamin C include many fruits and vegetables.

Vitamin E. Vitamin E completes the triumvirate of antioxidant vitamins that appear to confer protection against cardiovascular disease. Two major studies of health care professionals, done at Brigham and Women's Hospital and the Harvard School of Public Health in Boston, confirm other studies by the

World Health Organization that low levels of vitamin E are a more important predictor of ischemic heart disease than high cholesterol levels. This protective effect is seen with intake of more than 100 IUs per day. Vitamin E is the main fat-soluble antioxidant nutrient in the body. It lodges within the membranes inside and surrounding the cells, protecting the body against attack by singlet (unstable) oxygen and other free radicals that cause cell destruction. As mentioned earlier, singlet oxygen or other free-radical destruction of LDL cholesterol may be one of the early steps leading to atherogenesis and ultimately cardiovascular disease. Vitamin E, along with beta carotene and vitamin C, provides protection for both the water compartment and the fat compartment of our cells. This is necessary for the most complete protection against oxidative damage. Vitamin E also has a beneficial anticlotting effect on the blood. While a high-saturated-fat diet tends to cause blood cells to become sticky and clump together, vitamin E helps prevent this by causing the cells to disperse. This helps prevent blood clots from forming, an advantage for women past midlife who are at higher risk for stroke and heart attack.

Essential Fatty Acids. The supplemental use of Omega-3 fatty acids have certain protective effects against cardiovascular disease. In a number of medical studies, Omega-3 fatty acids have been shown to inhibit platelet cell aggregation (important in preventing clot formation) as well as relaxing and dilating the blood vessels. In addition, Omega-3 fatty acids lower the level of triglycerides; this is beneficial because elevated levels of triglycerides are a risk factor for coronary artery disease.

Omega-3 fatty acids are derived from certain fish oils such as mackerel, salmon and halibut, as well as certain plants such as flax seed, pumpkin seed and soybeans. While they can help lower the level of triglycerides, the benefits for reducing LDL cholesterol are not as clear cut. Also, because fish oil consumption can impair insulin secretion and increase blood glucose, fatty acid intake should be monitored in diabetics. Otherwise, the use of the Omega-3 fatty acids may be good for women wanting to prevent cardiovascular disease.

Breast Cancer

Vitamin A.   Beta carotene, the provitamin A found in fruits and vegetables, has been cited in a number of studies as being an important nutrient in breast cancer prevention. In the recent Nurses Health Study sponsored by Harvard University, which looked at the health and lifestyle habits of over 87,000 women, beta carotene indeed had a protective effect. Another recent study published in 1992 by the State University of New York compared 310 women having breast cancer to 316 women without the disease. The study found that the cancer-free group consumed many more beta carotene-containing fruits and vegetables than the women with breast cancer. In addition, The National Cancer Institute looked at 83 women with breast cancer and found that they had lower blood levels of beta carotene. Both beta carotene in supplemental form as well as abundant fresh fruits and vegetables should be included in your diet if you are concerned about breast cancer prevention.

Vitamin C.   In a 1991 review of 46 studies of the protective effect of vitamin C on cancer, the results of 33 studies showed that vitamin C helped safeguard against the development of many cancers; this included nonhormone-dependent breast cancer. Vitamin C did not appear to confer any protection against hormone-dependent (including estrogen-dependent) breast cancers.

Because fruits and vegetables are rich sources of both beta carotene and vitamin C, they are ideal sources of these nutrients. Women who wish to lower their cancer risk for all types of cancer (including certain breast cancers) may also want to use supplemental vitamin C.

Vitamin and Mineral Supplements for Women in Midlife

Good dietary habits are crucial for control of menopausal symptoms. Many women also need nutritional supplements in order to achieve higher levels of certain essential nutrients. Two formulas are included in this section—a general menopause formula and a vitamin and mineral formula for anemia due to premenopausal heavy menstrual flow. You may put these formulas together yourself by combining the individual nutrients. They provide excellent nutritional support for women during premenopausal years when heavy bleeding due to excessive estrogen levels and fibroids can be at their worst. It is also an excellent formula for women during their menopausal and post-menopausal years, providing complete nutritional support. Women with anemia due to heavy menstrual flow may also want to try the iron formula.

Women differ in their nutritional needs. If you take the recommended vitamin and mineral supplements, start at one-quarter to one-half the dose recommended and, if needed, slowly work your way up to the higher dose level. You may find that you do best with slightly more or less of certain ingredients. Do not exceed six to eight capsules per day without the supervision of your physician.

Take supplements with meals or a snack. Very rarely, a woman will have a digestive reaction, such as nausea or indigestion, to supplements. If this happens, stop all supplements, then resume by adding one nutrient at a time until you find the one that adversely affects you. Eliminate from the supplemental program any nutrient(s) to which you have a reaction, or find a different formula base for that nutrient and determine if it continues to have an ill effect. If you have any specific questions, ask a health care professional knowledgeable about nutrition.

Optimal Nutritional Supplementation for Menopause

Vitamins and Minerals	Daily Dosage
Vitamin A	5000 IU
Beta carotene (provitamin A)	5000 IU
Vitamin B complex	
B_1 (thiamine)	50 mg
B_2 (riboflavin)	50 mg

Vitamins and Minerals	Daily Dosage
B_3 (niacinamide)	50 mg
B_5 (pantothenic acid)	50 mg
B_6 (pyridoxine)	30 mg
B_{12} (cyanocobalamin)	50 mcg
Folic acid	400 mcg
Biotin	200 mcg
Choline	50 mcg
Inositol	50 mg
PABA	50 mg
Vitamin C (as ascorbic acid)	1000 mg
Vitamin D	400 IU
Bioflavonoids	800 mg
Rutin	200 mg
Vitamin E (d-alpha tocopherol acetate)	800 IU
Calcium	1200 mg
Magnesium	320 mg
Potassium	100 mg
Iron	27 mg
Zinc	15 mg
Iodine	150 mcg
Manganese	10 mg
Copper	2 mg
Selenium	25 mcg
Chromium	100 mcg
Bromelain	100 mcg
Papain	65 mg
Boron	3 mg

Instructions: If you use the LIFECYCLE formula, take two to eight tablets per day. Eight tablets are equivalent to the formula listed above.

Women's Daily Iron Formula

Vitamins, Minerals, Herbs	Daily Dosage
Iron	27 mg
Vitamin C	250 mg
Vitamin E (natural d-alpha)	30 IU
Vitamin B complex	
B_1 (thiamine)	7.5 mg
B_2 (riboflavin)	7.5 mg
B_6 (pyridoxine)	30 mg
B_5 (pantothenic acid)	50 mg
B_3 (niacinamide)	10 mg
B_{12} (cyanocobalamin)	250 mcg
Folic acid	400 mcg
Biotin	100 mcg
Choline bitartrate	5 mg
Inositol	5 mg
PABA	5 mg
Zinc	1.5 mg
Copper	250 mcg
Betaine HCL	10 mg
Chlorophyll	35 mg
Licorice root	25 mg
Red clover	25 mg
Yellow dock	25 mg

Instructions: If you use the LIFECYCLE formula, take one capsule per day. One capsule is equivalent to the above formula.

Food Sources of Vitamin A

Vegetables	*Fruits*	*Meat, Poultry,*
Carrots	Apricots	*Seafood*
Carrot juice	Avocado	Crab
Collard greens	Cantaloupe	Halibut
Dandelion greens	Mangoes	Liver—all types
Green onions	Papaya	Mackerel
Kale	Peaches	Salmon
Parsley	Persimmons	Swordfish
Spinach		
Sweet potatoes		
Turnip greens		
Winter squash		

Food Sources of Vitamin B Complex (including folic acid)

Vegetables and	Onions	*Grains*
Legumes	Peas	Barley
Alfalfa	Pinto beans	Bran
Artichoke	Romaine lettuce	Brown rice
Asparagus	Soybeans	Corn
Beets		Millet
Broccoli	*Meat, Poultry,*	Rice bran
Brussels sprouts	*Seafood*	Wheat
Cabbage	Egg yolk*	Wheat germ
Cauliflower	Liver*	
Garbanzo beans		*Sweeteners*
Green beans		Blackstrap molasses
Kale		
Leeks		
Lentils	*Eggs and meat should be from organic, range-fed	
Lima beans	stock fed on pesticide-free food.*	

Food Sources of Vitamin B6

Grains	Meat, Poultry, Fish, Seafood	Vegetables
Brown rice	Chicken	Asparagus
Buckwheat flour	Salmon	Beet greens
Rice bran	Shrimp	Broccoli
Rice polishings	Tuna	Brussels sprouts
Rye flour		Cauliflower
Wheat germ		Green peas
Whole wheat flour	Nuts and Seeds	Leeks
	Sunflower seeds	Sweet potato

Food Sources of Vitamin C

Fruits	Vegetables	Meat, Poultry, Fish, Seafood
Blackberries	Asparagus	Liver—all types
Black currants	Black-eyed peas	Pheasant
Cantaloupe	Broccoli	Quail
Elderberries	Brussels sprouts	Salmon
Grapefruit	Cabbage	
Grapefruit juice	Cauliflower	
Guava	Collards	
Kiwi fruit	Green onions	
Mango	Green peas	
Orange	Kale	
Orange juice	Kohlrabi	
Pineapple	Parsley	
Raspberries	Potato	
Strawberries	Rutabaga	
Sweet pepper	Tangerine	
Sweet potato		
Tomato		
Turnips		

Food Sources of Vitamin E

Vegetables	*Meats, Poultry, Fish, Seafood*	*Oils*
Asparagus	Haddock	Corn oil
Cucumber	Herring	Peanut oil
Green peas	Lamb	Safflower oil
Kale	Liver—all types	Sesame oil
	Mackerel	Soybean oil
Nuts and Seeds		Wheat germ oil
Almonds		
Brazil nuts	*Grains*	*Fruits*
Hazelnuts	Brown rice	Mango
Peanuts	Millet	

Food Sources of Essential Fatty Acids

Flax oil	Sunflower oil
Pumpkin oil	Grape oil
Soybean oil	Corn oil
Walnut oil	Wheat germ oil
Safflower oil	Sesame oil

Food Sources of Iron

Grains

Bran cereal (All Bran)

Bran muffin

Millet, dry

Oak flakes

Pasta, whole-wheat

Pumpernickel bread

Wheat germ

Legumes

Black beans

Black-eyed peas

Garbanzo beans

Kidney beans

Lentils

Lima bean

Pinto beans

Soybeans

Split peas

Tofu

Vegetables

Beets

Beet greens

Broccoli

Brussels sprouts

Corn

Dandelion greens

Green beans

Kale

Leeks

Spinach

Sweet potato

Swiss chard

Fruits

Apple juice

Avocado

Blackberries

Dates, dried

Figs

Prunes, dried

Prune juice

Raisins

Meat, Poultry, Seafood

Beef liver

Calves' liver

Chicken liver

Clams

Oysters

Sardines

Scallops

Trout

Nuts and Seeds

Almonds

Pecans

Pistachios

Sesame butter

Sesame seeds

Sunflower seeds

Food Sources of Calcium

Vegetables
Artichoke
Black beans
Black-eyed peas
Beet green
Broccoli
Brussels sprouts
Cabbage
Collards
Eggplant
Garbanzo beans
Green beans
Green onions
Kale
Kidney beans
Leeks
Lentils
Parsley
Parsnips
Pinto beans
Rutabaga
Soybeans
Spinach
Turnips
Watercress

Meat, Poultry, Fish, Seafood
Abalone
Beef
Bluefish
Carp
Crab
Haddock
Herring
Lamb
Lobster
Oysters
Perch
Salmon
Shrimp
Venison

Fruits
Blackberries
Black currants
Boysenberries
Orange
Pineapple juice
Prunes
Raisins
Rhubarb
Tangerine juice

Grains
Bran
Brown rice
Bulgar
Millet

Food Sources of Magnesium

Vegetables	Meat, Poultry, Fish, Seafood	Nuts and Seeds
Artichoke	Beef	Almonds
Black-eyed peas	Carp	Brazil nuts
Carrot juice	Chicken	Hazelnuts
Corn	Clams	Peanuts
Green peas	Cod	Pistachios
Leeks	Crab	Pumpkin seeds
Lima beans	Duck	Sesame seeds
Okra	Haddock	Walnuts
Parsnips	Herring	
Potato	Lamb	Fruits
Soybean sprouts	Mackerel	Avocado
Spinach	Oysters	Banana
Squash	Salmon	Grapefruit juice
Yams	Shrimp	Pineapple juice
	Snapper	Prunes
	Turkey	Papaya
		Raisins
		Grains
		Brown rice
		Millet
		Wild rice

Food Sources of Potassium

Vegetables	Meat, Poultry, Fish, Seafood	Nuts and Seeds
Asparagus	Bass	Almonds
Black-eyed peas	Beef	Brazil nuts
Beets	Carp	Chestnuts
Brussels sprouts	Cat fish	Hazelnuts
Carrot juice	Chicken	Macadamia nuts
Cauliflower	Cod	Peanuts
Corn	Duck	Pistachios
Garbanzo beans	Eel	Pumpkin seeds
Green beans	Flat fish	Sesame seeds
Kidney beans	Haddock	Sunflower seeds
Leeks	Halibut	Walnuts
Lentils	Herring	
Lima beans	Lamb	**Grains**
Navy beans	Lobster	Brown rice
Okra	Mackerel	Millet
Parsnips	Oysters	Wild rice
Peas	Perch	
Pinto beans	Pike	**Fruits**
Potato	Salmon	Apricots
Pumpkin	Scallops	Avocado
Soybean sprouts	Shrimp	Banana
Spinach	Snapper	Cantaloupe
Squash	Trout	Currants
Yams	Turkey	Figs
		Grapefruit juice
		Orange juice
		Papaya
		Pineapple juice
		Prune
		Raisins

13

Herbs for Menopause

$\mathcal{H}$erbs have a long and distinguished history for the treatment of female complaints. Plant-based remedies were our first real medicines; the history of their use spans thousands of years. An understanding of their healing properties was based on observation as well as trial and error. Valuable research on medicinal benefits of plants continues today, using modern scientific techniques of testing and analysis.

Herbs can help balance and expand the diet while optimizing nutritional intake. If you are interested in using herbs, try them as a part of your menopause-relief nutritional program.

Herbs that Relieve Symptoms of Menopause

This section provides information on herbs that can help relieve menopause-related symptoms. Many women have found helpful and effective herbal remedies for the relief of common menopausal symptoms. These remedies, along with a healthy diet, are a form of extended nutrition.

Heavy or Irregular Menstrual Bleeding

Heavy or irregular menstrual bleeding is a common problem experienced by women progressing into menopause. Luckily, many bioflavonoid-containing plants can help smooth out menstrual irregularities and reduce the quantity of blood lost during this time of hormonal instability. They do this in two ways. Plants containing bioflavonoids strengthen the capillaries and help prevent them from rupturing, thereby reducing blood loss. In addition, bioflavonoids are weakly estrogenic, as well as anti-estrogenic. Because they compete with estrogen precursors in the body for binding sites on enzymes, they help reduce your own levels of estrogen, which can be quite high during the menopause transition period. This reduces estrogen stimulation to the uterine lining, decreasing the amount of blood flow that can occur with menstruation.

There are many good plant sources of bioflavonoids because they are found in a wide variety of fruits and flowers. Bioflavonoids are also responsible for the striking colors of many plants. Good sources of bioflavonoids include citrus fruits, bilberries, cherries and grape skins. Bioflavonoids have also been found in red clover and in some clover strains in Australia. Many of these plants are available as herbal tinctures (liquid) or in capsules and can be taken in supplemental form.

Two herbs that women have traditionally used to stop excessive menstrual flow and postpartum hemorrhage are golden seal and shepherd's purse. Recent research studies have supported those claims. Golden seal contains a chemical called berberine that calms uterine muscular tension. (It has also been used to calm and soothe the digestive tract.) Shepherd's purse helps promote blood clotting and has been used to help stop menstrual bleeding. If your bleeding is excessive or irregular, consult your physician. This should be evaluated carefully by your physician and, if necessary, medical therapy should be instituted. Excessive and irregular bleeding can be dangerous and should never be allowed to continue without medical help. Women with a normal menstrual flow that is somewhat heavier may find the mild properties of herbs helpful for symptom relief.

Other herbs help prevent iron-deficiency anemia that can result from heavy menstrual flow during the early menopause period. These herbs provide good sources of non-heme iron. Outstanding examples are yellow dock and pau d'arco. Yellow dock is also used to help promote liver health which is important in the regulation of estrogen levels because the liver breaks down estrogen and prepares it for excretion from the body. When estrogen levels are too high, heavy menstrual bleeding can occur. Turmeric, or curcuma, is also used to promote liver health in traditional medicine. Recent research suggests that it has antibacterial properties. Turmeric is an herb often used for flavoring in traditional Indian dishes. Silymarin, or milk thistle, contains strong antioxidants that protect the liver from damage.

Hot Flashes, Night Sweats, Vaginal and Bladder Atrophy

Phytoestrogen plants abound in nature. These plants contain natural sources of estrogen, similar to that manufactured by our own body. Many of these plants can be used as an estrogen substitute by women who cannot or do not want to use estrogen in pharmacological dosages. For women who have pre-existing health problems such as migraine headaches or hypertension or who are sensitive to the dosages used in standard replacement therapy, phytoestrogen herbs provide a helpful alternative.

Compared with drug potencies, plant sources of estrogen are very weak. Bioflavonoids, the type of estrogen found in many plants, are only 1/50,000 as potent as stilbestrol. (Stilbestrol is a synthetic form of estrogen. Its use has been discontinued in women today due to its toxic effects in humans, but was in vogue several decades ago.) Other estrogen-containing plants such as fennel and anise, common licorice-flavored kitchen herbs, have been assayed as 1/400 the potency of estradiol, the main form of estrogen made by the ovaries. Because of their low potencies, estrogen-containing herbs tend to have a low potential for causing side effects, yet are quite effective in suppressing such common menopause symptoms as hot flashes and night sweats. They can even help build up the vaginal walls, which tend to become thin and atrophy due to estrogen deficiency. Other plant sources of estrogen and progesterone used in traditional herbology include dong quai, black cohosh, blue cohosh, unicorn root, false unicorn root, sarsaparilla and wild yam root.

Plants may also form the basis for the production of medical hormones. Many common plants such as soy beans and yams contain a preformed steroidal nucleus. Estrogen and progesterone can be synthesized from plants in relatively few steps; this has allowed sex hormones to become available commercially at reasonable cost.

Women who suffer from vaginal and bladder atrophy due to estrogen deficiency run the additional risk of increased incidence of infections in these tissues because they become more delicate and easily traumatized after menopause. Many herbs appear to have an ability to soothe, relieve irritation and reduce infection in the urinary tract; these include golden seal, uva ursi, blackberry root and wintergreen. Golden seal contains berberine, an alkaloid with antibiotic activity. It may also help to combat vaginitis due to yeast infections, a real problem for many postmenopausal women. Uva ursi contains arbutin, a urinary diuretic and anti-infective agent.

Menopause-related Insomnia

Passion flower has been found to elevate levels of the neurotransmitter serotonin. Serotonin is synthesized from tryptophan, an essential amino acid that has been shown in numerous medical studies to initiate restful sleep. Chamomile, an herb that makes delicate, tasty tea, is a good source of tryptophan. Valerian root has been used extensively in traditional herbal medicine as a sleep inducer and is widely used both in Europe and the United States as a gentle herbal remedy to help combat insomnia. Unfortunately, valerian has an unpleasant taste, which is more palatable when used in capsule form.

I have been very pleased with the benefits these herbs have brought to my patients suffering from menopause-related anxiety and insomnia. Many women with moderate to severe symptoms of hormonal deficiency wake up two to three times a night. If you suffer from menopause-related insomnia, you may need to make a fairly strong sedative tea such as hops or chamomile, using two or three tea bags instead of one. Start with a weaker tea and increase the potency slowly until you find the level that works best for you.

Many menopausal women also suffer from the unpleasant physical symptoms of tight, tense muscles in vulnerable areas of their bodies (neck, shoulders and jaw as well as the upper and lower back are common areas to store tension). Many of these relaxant herbs help relieve the muscle tension and spasm that often accompanies stress. Certain herbs such as valerian root, peppermint and chamomile are also effective in relieving stress-related indigestion and intestinal gas.

Menopause Anxiety, Irritability and Insomnia

Specific herbs can provide helpful relief for the emotional and sleep-deprivation symptoms of menopause. Plants such as valerian root, passion flower, hops, chamomile and skull-cap have a significant calming and restful effect on the central nervous system. (Other calming herbs include bay, balm, catnip, celery, motherwort, wild cherry and yarrow). They all promote emotional calm and well-being. With their mild sedative effect, they also promote restful sleep, a difficult state to induce in a woman suffering from menopause-related insomnia.

Menopause-related Fatigue and Depression

Menopausal women commonly suffer from depression and fatigue. Sometimes these symptoms co-exist with anxiety and irritability. Menopausal women with mood swings that vacillate between highs and lows often feel that they are on an emotional roller coaster.

A number of herbs can help a woman with depressed feelings and fatigue due to anxiety episodes. Herbs such as oat straw, ginger, ginkgo biloba, dandelion root and Siberian ginseng (eleutherococcus) have a stimulatory effect, improving energy and vitality. Women who use these herbs may note an increased ability to handle stress, as well as improved physical and mental capabilities. Some of the salutary effects may be due to the high levels of essential nutrients found in herbs. For example, dandelion root contains magnesium, potassium and vitamin E, while ginkgo contains high levels of bioflavonoids.

Siberian ginseng and ginger have been important traditional medicines in China and other countries for thousands of years. They have been reputed to increase longevity and decrease fatigue and weakness. These herbs boost immunity and strengthen the cardiovascular system. The bioflavonoids contained in ginkgo are extremely powerful antioxidants and help to combat fatigue by improving circulation to the brain. They also appear to have a strong affinity for the adrenal and thyroid gland and may help boost function in these essential glands. Oat straw can be used to relieve fatigue and weakness, especially when there has been an emotional upheaval.

In modern China, Japan and other countries, there is a great deal of interest in the pharmacological effects of these traditional herbs. Scientific studies are corroborating the medicinal effects of these plants.

Conditions Affected by Herbs

Osteoporosis, Heart Disease and Breast Disease

Herbs can provide a valuable source of minerals along with other foods in the diet. Certain plants such as kelp and other sea vegetables as well as dandelion root, horsetail and oat straw are good sources of calcium, magnesium and trace minerals needed for strong and healthy bones. Kelp and the other sea vegetables can be used as condiments to flavor food such as soups, casseroles and salads. The other herbs may be taken in capsule form as a supplement.

Garlic and ginger are two delicious herbs that are used commonly as flavoring agents. They are also tremendously beneficial in reducing risk of heart disease. These two plants should be used frequently as part of your preventative program if you have a strong family history of heart disease with early mortality (parents or siblings dying in their 50s or 60s of heart disease). They should also be used if you have any risk factors yourself, such as hypertension or elevated cholesterol. Both garlic and ginger have been researched for their ability to prevent aggregation or clotting of the blood. This is important for the prevention of strokes and heart attacks. In addition, both herbs help reduce cholesterol levels. Garlic has the additional benefit of reducing blood pressure.

If you find these foods too spicy for your taste buds, they can be used in capsule form or as a liquid tincture. Women using these herbs for cardiovascular disease prevention may want to eat several raw cloves of garlic a day or take as many as six capsules of the herb as a supplement. I also recommend as many as four capsules of ginger per day, if you do not use it as a food flavoring. These are maximum dosages; you may find that one to two capsules per day suit your needs better.

Many herbs show promise in the prevention or treatment of many human cancers, although their specific role in treating breast cancer is not clear. Herbs with possible anticancer activity include garlic, burdock root, alfalfa and a host of others. One herb in particular may hold some promise for breast cancer prevention. This is red clover, an herb traditionally used by several different cultures to treat cancer. Research done at the National Cancer Institute has found anticarcinogenic compounds in red clover, including several bioflavonoids, genistein and daidzein, which are both weakly estrogenic and anti-estrogenic. Women with a pre-existing breast cancer may want to check with their physician to see if red clover can be used safely as a nutritional adjunct to their regular medical program.

Herbal Formulas for Women in Midlife

Herbs are an effective means of balancing the diet and optimizing nutritional intake. Here are three herbal formulas that provide optimal nutritional support for women suffering from menopause-related complaints. Formula 1 can be used with general menopause complaints such as hot flashes and vaginal dryness due to hormonal deficiency. Formula 2 is very helpful for women with menopause-related fatigue, debility and weakness. Formula 3 can be used by women with menopause-related anxiety, irritability and insomnia.

You can purchase a commercial mixture or put together all three formulas yourself by mixing herbs in equal ratios.

Herbal Formula 1	Black cohosh
	Don quai
	False unicorn root
	Fennel
	Anise
	Blessed thistle
Herbal Formula 2	Ginger
	Oat straw
	Ginkgo biloba
	Siberian ginseng (eleutherococcus)
Herbal Formula 3	Valerian root
	Catnip
	Chamomile
	Hops

The herbs should be used in small amounts and taken with your meals in either capsule form or in a tea. If you buy a commercial product, do not take more than one to two capsules per day of the herbal mix. If you prefer to make a tea, simply empty the capsule into a cup of boiling water and let it steep for a few minutes. Do not drink more than one or two cups of the tea per day.

All foods have the potential for causing distress in some people and herbs are no exception. They should be discontinued immediately if you experience nausea, vomiting or diarrhea after use. These are the most common symptoms of intolerance. The herbs in my formulas are all recommended as being safe for human consumption, but rarely a woman may react adversely to various foods, including herbs. If you notice any symptoms that make you uncomfortable after using the herbs, discontinue them immediately.

Herbs for Menopause and Female Health Problems

Symptoms	Herbal Treatments
Heavy and irregular menstrual flow	Citrus fruit inner peel
	Cherry skins
	Grape skins
	Bilberry
	Red clover
	Golden seal
	Yellow dock
	Pau d'arco
	Turmeric
	Silymarin
Hot flashes, night sweats, vaginal and bladder atrophy	Citrus fruit inner peel
	Cherry skins
	Grape skins
	Anise
	Fennel
	Red clover
	Wild yam root
	Dong quai
	Black cohosh
	Unicorn root
	False unicorn root

Menopause insomnia and anxiety	Valerian root
	Passion flower
	Peppermint
	Catnip
	Chamomile
	Hops
Menopause, fatigue, tiredness and depression	Oat straw
	Ginger
	Dandelion root
	Siberian ginseng
	Blessed thistle
Menopause bladder and lower urinary tract symptoms	Golden seal
	Uva ursi
	Blackberry root
	Wintergreen
Osteoporosis	Kelp
	Dandelion root
	Horsetail
	Oat straw
Atherosclerosis	Garlic
	Ginger
Breast cancer	Red clover

Plants Used for Commercial Hormone Synthesis

Plant Source	Preformed Steroidal Nucleus
Soybean	Stigmasterol
Calabas bean	Ergosterol
Yeast	B-Sitosterol
Cereal grains	Diosgenin
Yams	Hecogenin
Sisal	

14

Stress Reduction for Menopause

$\mathcal{M}$enopause may be a time of mood swings and emotional upset for many women. This can occur both during the transition towards menopause and the early postmenopausal years. Often, these emotional changes are due to the instability in the female hormones, estrogen and progesterone, as they readjust to a new and lower level of equilibrium. Both estrogen and progesterone affect brain chemistry (progesterone has a sedative effect and estrogen acts as a brain stimulant); therefore, their fluctuating levels can wreak havoc on both mood and body. Emotional symptoms of menopause can include anxiety, irritability, emotional fragility, anger, depression, crying easily, and fatigue. Also, when hot flashes occur at night, they are often linked to insomnia.

Severity of these symptoms will vary amongst women due to differences in individual biochemistry as well as stressful and aggravating social factors. Some women go through menopause with no mood changes at all, feeling calm and relaxed. Other women have moderate to severe symptoms which can be incapacitating, interfering with their quality of life.

For many women, the social and cultural factors occurring around the time of menopause can be as significant as hormonal changes in determining their emotional state. Menopause can be a time of loss, with parents dying or ill, children leaving home, and careers or marriages ending. Often, the old familiar guideposts that have provided stability during the first half of life disappear, leaving a woman feeling lost. On the positive side, it can also be a time of rebirth for the woman and a time of forging or solidifying her own identity. The rebirth process can be difficult and take years to complete. Thus, for many women, the combination of hormonal and biochemical changes plus the social factors can be quite difficult to handle.

Some women require counseling and medication in order to cope with menopause-related emotional symptoms. All women can benefit from self-help techniques such as stress reduction and relaxation exercises. Since the physical, chemical, and social changes are unavoidable, practicing these types of techniques on a regular basis can help bring a sense of peace, calm and stability to your life.

The rest of this chapter is divided into three sections: stress-reduction exercises you can use for general relaxation, for specific premenopause symptoms, and for menopause-related symptoms. Each section contains many different types of exercises so that you can find the ones that work best for you. Try the relaxation techniques that pertain to your symptoms; enjoy the many emotional and physical benefits they bring over time.

Before you begin the exercises, separate yourself physically and mentally from your normal day-to-day environment. At home, find a quiet place where you can be alone. At work, close the door to your office while you take a relaxation break. Many women find that quiet background music promotes a sense of peace as they exercise. Classical music or environmental sounds such as ocean waves or the sound of rain can be very relaxing. In some exercises you sit upright in a comfortable position; in others, the exercises are performed while lying on your back. In either case, your arms and legs should be uncrossed. It is important that your clothes be loose and comfortable. Before you begin each exercise, close your eyes and take a few deep breaths in and out. This will help quiet your mind and remove your thoughts from the tasks of the day.

General Relaxation Exercises

I recommend beginning each stress-reduction session with some general relaxation exercises. These exercises will help you transition from your normal busy schedule and day-to-day activities. As you begin to unwind, you will become more receptive to the specific stress-reduction exercises for premenopause and menopause symptoms. The general relaxation exercises also promote good health and well-being for the entire body. You may want to practice them when you feel like taking a quick break during the busy times of the day. The exercises will give you a pick-me-up when your energy starts to wane and your mental edge begins to feel dull. They should rapidly begin to energize and revitalize you.

Exercise 1: Deep Abdominal Breathing

Abdominal breathing is a very important technique for inducing a state of peace and relaxation as well as improving energy and vitality. These can be very valuable goals for women when their physical and emotional well-being is impaired by the chemical and physiological instability of midlife. Deep, slow breathing brings adequate oxygen, the fuel for metabolic activity, to all the tissues of your body. In contrast, the rapid, shallow breathing that occurs during times of stress decreases the oxygen supply, keeping you tired and energy-depleted. Deep breathing helps release tension and anxiety and relaxes the entire body. It also helps balance many other important physiological processes such as pulse rate and hormonal output, thereby improving health.

- Lie flat on your back with your knees pulled up, keeping your feet slightly apart. Try to breathe in and out through your nose.

- Inhale deeply. As you breathe in, allow your stomach to relax so the air flows into your abdomen. Your stomach should balloon out as you breathe in. Visualize your lungs filling with air so your chest swells out.

- Imagine that the air you breathe is filling your body with energy.

- Exhale deeply. As you breathe out, let your stomach and chest collapse. Image the air being pushed out, first from your abdomen and then from your lungs.

- Repeat this exercise 10 times.

Exercise 2: Focusing

- Sit upright in a comfortable position.

- Hold a small, sentimental object in the palm of your hand.

- Focus all of your attention on this object as you inhale and exhale deeply for one to two minutes. Don't let any other thoughts enter your mind.

- At the end of this time, notice your breathing. You should find that it has slowed down and is calm. You will probably feel a sense of peacefulness and a decrease in any stress or tension that you started with when beginning this exercise.

The next three exercises help you identify your areas of muscle tension and then teach you how to release this tension. This is an important sequence for women in transition, menopause, or postmenopause who suffer from heavy menstrual flow, blood clots, recurrent menstrual cramps, low back pain, or vaginal and bladder atrophy. Many of these symptoms increase when women localize tension and stress to their pelvic area. Chronically tight and tense muscles in the low back and pelvic region can intensify menopause symptoms. Tense muscles tend to have decreased blood circulation and oxygenation, and may accumulate an excess of waste products, such as carbon dioxide and lactic acid.

Interestingly, many women (and men) tend to tighten and contract certain muscle groups as a habitual reaction to strong emotional patterns. For example, if a person has difficulty expressing feelings verbally, the neck muscles may become chronically tight. A person with repressed anger may have chest pain and tight chest muscles. Many women tend to tighten the pelvis and lower abdominal muscles as a stress response to a variety of work, relationship, and sexual stresses. Usually, the tensing of pelvic muscles is an unconscious response that develops over many years and sets up the emotional patterning that triggers pelvic tension-related symptoms. For example, when a woman has uncomfortable feelings about sex or a particular sexual partner, she may tighten these muscles when engaging in or even thinking about sex. Tense muscles can affect a woman's moods, making her more "uptight" and irritable.

Movement through stretching or exercise is one effective way of breaking up these habitual patterns of muscle tensing and contracting. When muscles are loose and limber, a woman will feel more relaxed and in a better mood. Tension and stress fades away, replaced by a sense of expansiveness. The following exercise will help you release tension in your tight muscle groups.

Exercise 3: Discovering Muscle Tension

- Lie on your back in a comfortable position. Allow your arms to rest comfortably at your sides, palms down, on the surface next to you.

- Raise your right arm straight up and hold it elevated for 15 seconds.

- Notice if your forearm feels tight and tense or if the muscles are soft and pliable.

- Let your arm drop down and relax. The arm muscles will relax, too.

- As you lie quietly, notice any other parts of your body that feel tense, muscles that feel tight and sore. You may feel a constant dull aching in certain muscles. Tense muscles block blood flow and cut off the supply of nutrients to the tissues. In response to the poor oxygenation, the muscle produces lactic acid, which further increases muscular discomfort.

- Release the tension in any tense or aching muscles.

Exercise 4: Progressive Muscle Relaxation

- Lie on your back in a comfortable position. Allow your arms to rest at your sides, palms down, on the surface next to you.

- Inhale slowly and deeply through your nose and exhale slowly through your mouth.

- Clench your hands into fists and hold them tightly for 15 seconds. Visualize your fists contracting, becoming tighter and tighter. As you do this, relax the rest of your body.

- Let your hands relax. As you relax, visualize a golden light flowing into the entire body, making all your muscles soft and pliable.

- Now, tense and relax the following parts of your body in this order: face, shoulders, back, stomach, pelvis, legs, feet, and toes. Hold each part tensed for 15 seconds and then relax your body for 30 seconds before going on to the next part.

- Finish the exercise by shaking your hands and imagining the remaining tension flowing out of your fingertips.

Exercise 5: Release of Muscle Tension and Anxiety

- Lie in a comfortable position. Allow your arms to rest at your sides, palms down. Inhale and exhale slowly and deeply with your eyes closed.

- Become aware of your feet, ankles, and legs. Notice whether parts of your body have any muscle tension or tightness. If so, how does the tense part of your body feel? Is it in a viselike grip, knotted, cold, numb? Do you notice any strong feelings, such as hurt, upset, or anger in that part of your body? Breathe into that part of your body until you feel it relax. Release any anxious feelings with your breathing, continuing until they begin to decrease in intensity and fade.

- Next, move your awareness into your hips, pelvis, and lower back. Note any tension or anxious feelings located in that part of your body. Breathe into your hips and pelvis until you feel them relax. Release any negative emotions as you breathe in and out.

- Focus on your abdomen and chest. Notice any anxious feelings located in this area and let them drop away as you breathe in and out. Continue to release any upsetting feelings located in your abdomen or chest.

- Finally, focus on your head, neck, arms, and hands. Note any tension in this area and release it. With your breathing, release any negative feelings blocked in this area until they disappear.

- When you have finished releasing tension throughout the body, continue deep breathing and relaxing for another minute or two. At the end of this exercise, you should feel lighter and more energized.

Stress-reduction Exercises for Premenopause

The premenopause time can be marked by symptoms of easily triggered feelings such as anxiety, irritability, mood swings, and depression. Physical symptoms include menstrual periods becoming irregular and menstrual flow either more excessive or diminished. In addition, fibroid tumors that have a potential for growing into large ovarian cysts are fairly common and PMS symptoms intensify. Clearly, many women experience this as a stressful time.

The next two exercises help create an easier and less traumatic menopause period by promoting a positive body–mind interaction. Since the mind, in part, affects the body's level of functioning, positive messages and visual pictures about your changing body can promote optimal health and well-being during this time. Positive mental messages can help reduce symptoms and smooth out the stress inherent in this time of change.

Exercise 6: Affirmations for Premenopause

Affirmations are positive statements that describe how you want your body to be. They are very important because they align your mind with your body in a positive way. Affirmations accomplish this through the power of suggestion. Your state of health is determined, in part, by the thousands of mental messages you send yourself each day. You can aggravate your premenopause symptoms such as excessive bleeding and cramps due to fibroid tumors or anovulatory periods (menstrual cycles when you don't produce progesterone), or even PMS symptoms, with negative thoughts. When your body believes it is sick, it behaves accordingly. It is essential that you cultivate a positive belief system and a positive body image as part of your healing program. It is not enough to follow an excellent diet and a vigorous exercise routine when you are in the process of reducing premenopausal symptoms. You must also tell your body that it is a well, fully functional system. I have seen people remain ill by sabotaging their healing program when they send themselves a barrage of negative messages.

- Sit in a comfortable position. Repeat the following affirmations, repeating three times those that are particularly important to you.

- My female system is strong and healthy.

- My hormonal levels are perfectly balanced and regulated.

- My body chemistry is healthy and balanced.

- I go through my monthly menstrual cycle with ease and comfort.

- My menstrual flow self-regulates. I have a moderate, comfortable menstrual flow.

- I never spot between menstrual cycles.

- I am free of blood clots.

- My menstrual cycle comes at the right time each month. I have a regular cycle.

- My vaginal muscles, cervix, and uterus are relaxed and comfortable.

- My uterus is normal size and shape.

- My menstrual flow leaves my body easily and effortlessly each month.

- My body feels wonderful as I start each monthly period.

- I barely know that my body is getting ready to menstruate.

- I feel wonderful each month before I menstruate.

- My ovaries and uterus are healthy.

- My thyroid gland is healthy and helps regulate my menstrual flow.

- My low back muscles feel supple and pliable with each menstrual cycle.

- I am relaxed and at ease as my period approaches.

- I desire a well-balanced and healthful diet.

- I eat only the foods that are good for my female body.

- It is a real pleasure to take good care of my body.

- I do the level of exercise that keeps my body healthy and supple.

- I handle stress easily and in a relaxed manner.

- I love my body; I feel at ease in my body.

- I create perfect health and well-being within my body.

Exercise 7: Visualizations
for Premenopause

Visualization exercises help you create the mental blueprint for a healthier body. This powerful technique can stimulate the positive chemical and hormonal changes in your body, helping achieve the desired outcome. Through positive visualization, you are imaging your body the way you want it to function and to be. The body can modify its chemical and hormonal output in response to this technique and move toward a state of improved health. As a result, you may find this technique useful for reducing the symptoms that occur during the premenopause time.

Women (and men) with many types of illnesses have used visualization to their benefit. Visualization was pioneered by Carl Simonton, M.D., a cancer radiation therapist, who used this technique with his patients. Instead of seeing their cancer as a "big destructive monster," he had his patients see their immune system as big white knights or white sharks attacking the small and insignificant cancer cells and destroying them (instead of the other way around). In a substantial number of cases, he saw his patient's health improve. In this visualization exercise, I utilize an "erasure" image that helps you see any fibroids, ovarian cysts, old scar tissue, or other accumulated "wear and tear" on your body melt away and disappear. Then, these stressed areas are replaced by positive visualizations consistent with reproductive health and well-being. Skip any parts of the exercise that do not pertain to you.

- Sit in a comfortable position.

- Close your eyes. Begin to breathe deeply, slowly inhaling through your nose and exhaling through your mouth. Feel your body begin to relax.

- Imagine that you can look, as if through a magic mirror, deep inside your body.

- First, focus on any areas of your reproductive tract that you sense contain areas of damage or scarring. These can include tissue damage from old infections or areas of endometriosis.

- Next, imagine a large eraser—the kind used to erase chalk marks—entering into your pelvic area. See this eraser rubbing out areas of tissue damage or old scar tissue. See these areas begin to loosen, shrink, and finally disappear.

- Then look at your female organs. See your uterus: it is an attractive pink color. Your uterus is relaxed and supple. Any fibroid tumors are melting away as you look at them. Your uterus is becoming its normal size and shape. Your uterus has good blood circulation.

- Now, see the lining of your uterus. It is a lush, blood-rich cushion of tissue.

- Imagine that your uterus is currently in the state that occurs immediately before your menstrual cycle begins. The blood vessels in the lining of the uterus begin to constrict. See them become coiled and narrow. Visualize them as they begin to release the perfect amount of blood from the uterine lining.

- The blood flows out of the uterus in a moderate, regular flow. See the blood leave the uterus in a steady, healthy manner.

- See the uterine lining slough off into the blood flow so the uterus can prepare for the next month's cycle.

- Visualize your ovaries and fallopian tubes as they connect into the sides of the uterus. Your ovaries are shaped like almonds. See any cysts on the ovaries melt away until they disappear. Your ovaries are shiny, pink, and healthy looking. See them put out healthy levels of your female hormones, estrogen and progesterone. Your ovaries are perfectly regulated and function well each month.

- Look at your abdominal and low back muscles. They are soft and pliable with a healthy muscle tone. They are relaxed and free of tension during your menstrual period. Your abdomen is flat and your fluid balance is perfect in your pelvic area.

- Look at your entire body and enjoy the sense of peace and calm running through your body. You feel wonderful.

- Now stop visualizing the scene and go back to deep breathing.

- Open your eyes and feel very good. Visualizing these scenes should take several minutes. Be sure to linger on any images that particularly please you.

Stress-reduction Exercises for Menopause

While the physical and emotional symptoms of menopause are primarily due to the rapid and sustained drop in the estrogen and progesterone levels, stress can also play a significant role in both triggering and intensifying menopause symptoms. For example, hot flashes, the most common symptom of menopause, frequently occur when women are engaged in an activity or situation about which they feel emotionally tense or nervous. Many of my patients report an increase in the frequency of hot flashes when they have to give a speech, do a presentation in front of a group, mix at large social gatherings, or complete an important task on a tight time schedule. Thus, how well you manage stress can have tremendous repercussions on the ease or severity of your menopause symptoms. Positive beliefs and visualizations about your body during this time can decrease the level of stress hormones, thereby promoting healthier chemical and physiological responses on the body. This will help reduce the intensity of menopause-related symptoms.

In this section, I have included relaxation exercises to help you master your level of stress more effectively as a means of reducing menopausal symptoms. Other exercises have been included to help you develop a positive body image during this time of great change, *in effect, using your mind to create the healthy body you would like to have during your menopausal and post-menopausal years.*

Exercise 8: Meditation

Meditation requires you to sit quietly and engage in a simple and repetitive activity. By emptying your mind, you give yourself a rest. The metabolism of your body slows down. Meditating gives your mind a break from tension and worry. It is a useful exercise to do during early menopause, when every little stress is magnified by the drop in hormone levels that your body is experiencing. After meditating, you may find your mood greatly improved and your ability to handle everyday stress enhanced. This quieting of the body and mind can be very helpful to menopausal women who find their symptoms intensified by even little day-to-day stresses.

- Sit or lie in a comfortable position.

- Close your eyes and breathe deeply. Let your breathing be slow and relaxed.

- Focus all your attention on your breathing. Notice the movement of your chest and abdomen, in and out.

- Block out all other thoughts, feelings, and sensations. If you feel your attention wandering, bring it back to your breathing.

- As you inhale, say the word "peace" to yourself; as you exhale, say the word "relax." Draw out the pronunciation of the word so that it lasts for the entire breath. The word "peace" sounds like p-e-e-a-a-a-c-c-c-e-e-e. The word "relax" sounds like r-r-r-e-e-e-l-l-l-a-a-x-x. Repeating these words as you breathe will help you concentrate.

- Repeat this exercise until you feel calm and restful.

Exercise 9: Healing Meditation

This exercise induces a sense of peace and calm through a series of positive images. I have included a series of beautiful and peaceful images that will help create a positive mental state during times when life simply seems too frantic or busy. This meditation allows you to withdraw from your usual environment by going within yourself to find a place of healing. When you return, you will feel refreshed, better able to meet the daily life challenges many midlife women must deal with in addition to the physical stress of menopause.

This meditation is based on the fact that our mind and body are inextricably linked. When we visualize a beautiful scene where our body is being healed, we stimulate positive chemical and hormonal changes that can reduce pain, discomfort and irritability. Likewise, if you visualize a negative scene such as a fight with a spouse or a boss, the negative mental picture can trigger a chemical output in your body that exaggerates menopause-related symptoms. The axiom "you are what you think" is quite true. I have seen the power of positive thinking, and I advise my patients that healing the body is much harder if the mind is full of angry or fearful images. Healing meditations, when practiced on a regular basis, can be a powerful healing tool. If you enjoy this form of meditation, try designing your own exercises with images that make you feel good.

- Lie on your back in a comfortable position. Inhale through your nose and exhale slowly and deeply through your mouth.

- Visualize a beautiful green meadow full of lovely fragrant flowers. In the middle of this meadow is a golden temple. See the temple emanating peace and healing.

- Visualize yourself entering this temple. You are the only person inside. It is still and peaceful. As you stand inside, you feel a healing energy fill every pore of your body with a warm, golden light. Every cell in your body that is in need of repair and healing is nourished by this light. This energy feels like a healing balm that relaxes you totally. All stress dissolves and fades from your mind. You feel totally at ease. Remain in this temple for as long as you wish.

- When you are ready to leave, open your eyes and continue your slow, deep breathing for a few more cycles.

The next two exercises will help you gain mastery over stress by learning to shrink it or even erase it with your mind. Stress is then put in a much more manageable and realistic perspective. These two exercises will also help engender a sense of power and mastery, thereby reducing nervous tension and restoring a sense of calm.

Often situations and beliefs look large and insurmountable, making us feel nervous and tense. In this scenario, women tend to feel tiny and helpless while the people or situations generating the stress appear huge and problems seem unsolvable. These feelings are often intensified during menopause when decline in hormonal levels makes our coping ability more tenuous. Situations that wouldn't normally cause women distress can create irritability, tearfulness, and a variety of other emotional responses. Some women even create mental pictures that produce feelings of helplessness.

Exercise 10: Shrinking Stress

- Sit or lie in a comfortable position. Breathe slowly and deeply.

- Visualize a situation, person or even a belief ("I can't handle more tension with my boss" or "I don't want to give that public speech") that makes you feel upset or tense.

- As you do this, you might see a person's face, a place where you're uncomfortable or simply a dark cloud. Where do you see this stressful picture? Is it above you, to one side, or in front of you? How does it look? Is it large or small, dark or light? Does it have certain colors?

- Now slowly begin to shrink the stressful picture. Continue to see the stressful picture shrinking until it is so small that it can be held in your hands. As you hold your hand out in front of you, place the picture in the palm of your hand.

- If the stressor has a characteristic sound (such as a voice or traffic noise), hear it becoming softer. As it continues to diminish, the voice or sound becomes almost inaudible.

- Now the stressful picture is so small it can fit on the tip of a finger. Watch it shrink from there until it finally turns into a little dot and disappears.

- Often this exercise causes feelings of amusement, as well as relaxation, as the feared stressor shrinks, becomes less intimidating, and finally disappears.

Exercise 11: Erasing Stress

- Sit or lie in a comfortable position. Breathe slowly and deeply.

- Visualize a situation, person or even a belief ("I'm worried about losing my job" or "I'm uncomfortable mixing with other people at parties") that causes you to feel upset or tense.

- As you do this you might see a specific person, a place, or simply shapes and colors. Where do you see this stressful picture? Is it below you, to the side, in front of you? How does it look? Is it large or small, dark or light, or does it have a specific color?

- Imagine that a large eraser—the kind used to erase chalk marks—has floated into your hand. Actually feel and see the eraser in your hand. Take the eraser and begin to rub it over the area where the stressful picture is located. As the eraser rubs out the stressful picture, the picture begins to fade, shrink, and finally disappear. When you can no longer see the stressful picture, simply continue to focus on your deep breathing for another minute, inhaling and exhaling slowly and deeply.

Exercise 12: Glandular Breathing

Optimal endocrine function is very important for the reduction and prevention of menopausal symptoms. Healthy endocrine function is also needed for disease resistance, vitality, and energy. During menopause, the decline in output of female hormones estrogen and progesterone is less severe when the glands regulating the hormones are healthy. In fact, small amounts of female hormones continue to be secreted from the ovaries, adrenals, and fat tissue even after menopause.

This exercise helps stimulate and energize your endocrine glands through the use of color breathing. When you direct your breath into the endocrine glands and visualize them being infused by color, the glands are stimulated in a beneficial way. The use of color breathing expands the glands' electromagnetic field. In this exercise, the color red is used. Research studies with red light have shown that this color stimulates both endocrine and immune function.

- Sit upright in a chair, your arms at your sides, palms up. Imagine a large balloon filled with red color above your head. This is a bright, vibrant tone of red that sparkles with energy. As you inhale deeply, see yourself popping this balloon and releasing the red color. Allow the red color to flow into your head and concentrate in the hypothalamus, a gland located at the base of the brain. As the hypothalamus begins to overflow with color, exhale and breathe the red out of your lungs, filling the air around you.

- As you inhale again, breathe the bright red color into your pituitary, an important endocrine gland located in your brain, right below the hypothalamus. Fill the pituitary with this color until it overflows. Then exhale deeply.

- As you continue to inhale the bright red color, let it flow into your thyroid gland, located in your neck, then into your thymus gland, located in the middle of your chest. Finally, let the color energize your adrenal glands, located in the middle of your back above the kidneys, and your ovaries, located in the pelvis. When you finish this exercise, relax for a few minutes, breathing in and out slowly and deeply.

The next two exercises present you with a series of affirmations or positive statements that will help you to create an excellent state of health as well as facilitate the practice of a healthy lifestyle. During the menopause years and beyond, it is not enough to exercise vigorously and follow a healthy diet; it is also important to like your body and think positive thoughts as you go through the changes related to menopause. This is because your state of health is determined by the interaction between your mind and body, by the thousands of messages you send yourself each day with your thoughts. You can aggravate your menopause symptoms with negative thoughts because when your body believes it is sick, it behaves accordingly.

You may find when repeating certain affirmations that you have negative feelings about your body and menopause; these correspond to deeply held beliefs about your body that you would like to change. This exercise is very effective in helping change negative, unhappy thoughts to positive thoughts of self-love and acceptance. Doing this exercise on a regular basis will help you like your body more as you go through the changes of menopause. You may want to emphasize certain affirmations while deleting others. Writing each affirmation three times can also be very effective.

Exercise 13: Affirmations for Menopause

- Sit in a comfortable position. Repeat the following affirmations three times.

- I go through menopause easily and effortlessly.

- My body is healthy and strong during my menopause transition.

- My body becomes healthier each day.

- My hormones are perfectly balanced and regulated.

- My body chemistry is healthy and balanced.

- My female system is strong and healthy.

- My female organs are full of health and vitality.

- My body self-regulates its temperature control effectively.

- My skin temperature feels comfortable all the time.

- I sleep well every night.

- My vagina is moist and elastic, with good circulation.

- I have sexual relations as often as I desire.

- My mood is calm and relaxed.

- I handle stress easily and effortlessly

- My breasts are healthy and full of vitality.

- My thyroid is healthy and full of vitality.

- My bones and joints are strong and healthy.

- I feel wonderful as I go through menopause.

- I love my body.

Exercise 14: Menopause Lifestyle Affirmations

- Menopause is a beautiful time of growth and change for me.

- Menopause is presenting me with many opportunities to make wonderful and positive life changes.

- I take excellent care of myself during this time of change.

- I love to nurture myself.

- I take time each day to relax and enjoy myself.

- I practice the relaxation methods that I enjoy.

- I am enjoying my life more and more. My life brings me pleasure.

- I do my work and activities in a relaxed and comfortable way.

- I enjoy the company of my family and friends. They give me pleasure.

- I eat a well-balanced and healthful diet.

- I eat the foods that keep my body strong and healthy.

- I enjoy eating the foods that are delicious and full of healthy vitamins and minerals.

- As I get older, I am becoming stronger and healthier.

- I am full of vigor and vitality.

- Each day I practice the self-help methods that I enjoy. My life is fun and exciting.

Exercise 15: Visualizations for Menopause

This exercise uses visual pictures to help you achieve a more positive body image. It can help you create a mental blueprint of how you would like your body to look and function during menopause and beyond. Positive visualizations can help your body become healthier through creating a positive system of beliefs about your health. As you see your body radiating health and vitality, you stimulate chemical changes in your body to help create this condition.

In addition, positive visualization helps modify your behavior so that you can create the body pictures you like. You are more likely to choose the foods and nutrients as well as practice the exercises and self-care techniques when you practice the visualizations.

- Close your eyes. Begin to breathe deeply. Inhale and exhale slowly. Feel your body begin to relax.

- Imagine that you can look inside your body at your vital organs.

- Look at your female organs. They are full of energy and vitality. Your ovaries, uterus, and vagina are very healthy. They have an attractive pink color. Nutrients and oxygen flow freely to them and they release their waste products from your body. Your vagina is moist, pink, and healthy. It is elastic and expandable. You are able to enjoy a healthy and active sex life.

- Look at your breasts. The tissue is smooth, without lumps or masses. They feel comfortable when you touch them.

- Look at your thyroid (the gland below your Adam's apple in your neck). It has a healthy size and texture. It regulates your metabolism perfectly and functions normally.

- Look at your bones. They are strong and sturdy. They are full of calcium and other essential nutrients.

- Now, see your face. It is smooth and relaxed. It has a smile. You feel in command of yourself. You do not feel anxious, irritable, or depressed. Your mood is wonderful. As you look at yourself in the mental mirror, you know you can handle any problems that come along competently and with ease.

- Your skin is smooth and moist. Touch your face and hands. You take wonderful care of your skin by using moisturizers, sunscreens, and limiting your sun exposure. Your skin looks lovely.

- Look at your entire body and enjoy the feeling of energy and optimism that is running through you. You are very calm and peaceful.

- Now stop visualizing the scene and return to deep breathing.

- You open your eyes and feel very good.

- Visualizing this scene should take about forty-five seconds to one minute, longer if you choose to linger with a particular image. A visualization is successful when it allows you to change your feelings about a particular situation.

How to Choose the Right Stress-reduction Exercises

This chapter has introduced you to many different ways to reduce menopause-related tension and stress and has taught you how to use mental techniques to improve your state of health. Try each exercise that pertains to your symptoms at least once. Then find the combination that works best for you. Doing the exercises you enjoy most should take no longer than 10 to 20 minutes. Ideally, do the exercises daily. Over time, they will help you handle stress better and relax more easily. They will also help you change negative thoughts and feelings about menopause into positive, self-nurturing ones.

15

Physical Exercise and Menopause

$\mathcal{M}$any menopausal women neglect engaging in physical activity on a regular basis. In fact, nearly 17 percent of women are completely inactive, never exercising at all. This is unfortunate because exercise is one of the most beneficial self-help activities that a menopausal woman can do. A regular exercise program will help relieve and prevent common menopause symptoms including hot flashes, vaginal and bladder atrophy, emotional changes, and mood swings. In addition, physical activity can help prevent the longer-term problems associated with hormonal withdrawal and aging, such as bone loss, heart disease, and changes in weight and appearance. Many of the signs associated with aging actually result from physical inactivity. A sedentary lifestyle with little walking, lifting, or stretching causes poor circulation, shortness of breath, joint and muscle stiffness, fatigue and depression.

Treating Specific Menopause Symptoms with Exercise

Exercise should play a part in a good menopause self-help program. Let's examine how exercise can decrease your specific menopausal symptoms and improve your health.

Hot Flashes and Night Sweats

Women vary greatly in how they experience hot flashes in early menopause. Interestingly, the frequency and severity of hot flashes are not simply due to each woman's physiological programming (although this is certainly an important determinant). Many lifestyle factors also affect how severe the hot flash symptoms will be. Emotional stress and use of high-stress foods such as alcohol, coffee and chocolate can play an important role in triggering hot flashes. Luckily, both of these factors can be modified through good lifestyle habits. Exercise in particular can help reduce hot flashes for many women.

During their early menopausal years, many women find that they are more sensitive to everyday life stresses. Situations such as doing a presentation in front of a group, mixing with other people at social gatherings, or dealing with (or even thinking about) emotionally-charged family issues can bring on a series of hot flashes in susceptible women. Exercise practiced on a regular basis (at least three times a week for a half hour) can be the perfect remedy for discharging stress. In one study of the effect of aerobic exercise on hot flashes, 55 percent of the women reported a decrease in the severity of hot flashes. Their estrogen levels also rose following the exercise session. This link between estrogen levels and exercise emphasizes the importance of regular physical activity.

As well as elevating estrogen levels, exercise can help reduce the intensity of fight-or-flight stress response, which can be triggered by any situation that appears to be potentially dangerous or frightening. This response is mediated by the sympathetic nervous system which speeds up and heightens physiological functions we're normally unaware of, such as heart rate, skeletal muscle tension, and output of adrenal and thyroid hormones, all adjustments that allow a quick response to a threatening situation.

Unfortunately, many menopausal women may be in a state of constant nervous tension due to both the many social issues that occur during this time of change, as well as to their body's changing hormones and physiology. This can put women in a constant state of panic so they react to small stresses in the same way they would to real emergencies.

Exercise can help reduce hot flashes by providing an alternative way to discharge tension without harming your personal relationships or your body. After physical exercise, both the body and mind are calm, as physiological parameters including breathing and heart rate return to a more healthful resting level. The life problems and issues that trigger hot flashes often seem more manageable after a good exercise workout.

Exercise can also help reduce intake of frequently used addictive foods, alcohol and caffeine-containing coffee, tea, and chocolate, all of which can trigger hot flashes. Often those foods are overconsumed as a way to handle stress or as a pick-up to boost energy. Women can consciously substitute regular exercise in place of more harmful ways of dealing with stress or low energy states, thereby reducing the frequency of their hot flashes as an added benefit. In addition, an exercise program practiced three to five times a week is a positive habit that provides many health benefits in addition to reducing hot flashes.

Vaginal and Bladder Atrophy

Vaginal and bladder changes, such as thinning of the mucosa and loss of elasticity, trouble many menopausal women. These changes can lead to soreness and irritation of the vagina, urethra, and bladder, as well as pain during intercourse. In addition, recurrent bladder and vaginal infections are common. While these problems are due primarily to the decrease in female hormones needed to stimulate healthy tissue in this area, poor blood circulation and muscle tone in the pelvic area can also contribute to vaginal and bladder symptoms. This can be helped tremendously by regular physical activity, particularly when the pelvic muscles are involved.

One of the best types of physical exercise is sexual activity, which stimulates vaginal lubrication, good blood circulation to the vagina, and rhythmic movement of the pelvic muscles.

Studies have shown that women who continue to be sexually active after menopause (with at least one sexual encounter per week) either through sexual intercourse or masturbation tend to have fewer signs of vaginal aging. There is less vaginal shrinkage and loss of elasticity because the tissue is being gently stretched on a regular basis. In addition, women who remain sexually active tend to secrete higher levels of androgens (the male hormones) from their ovaries after menopause, although estrogen levels are unaffected. Interestingly enough, it is the small amounts of androgens that women secrete, rather than estrogen, that are responsible for maintaining libido or sexual desire.

Even nonsexual touching can improve circulation to the pelvic area through massage or gentle touching of the whole body which promotes muscle relaxation and improves circulation. Couples can give much pleasure to each other through learning simple massage techniques; single women can exchange massages with friends.

General aerobic exercise will help promote better muscle tone and blood circulation to the pelvic area. Physical exercise such as walking, tennis, or low-impact aerobics causes a vigorous pumping action of the skeletal muscles throughout the body, including the pelvis. This brings blood flow, oxygenation, and needed nutrients to the muscles in this area; it also helps remove waste products of metabolism, such as carbon dioxide and lactic acid, to maintain healthy vaginal and bladder tissues.

Local pelvic area exercises improve bladder control, vaginal elasticity, and can increase sexual pleasure. One set of exercises was developed by Dr. Arnold Kegel in the 1940s. The Kegel exercises strengthen the muscles that surround the urethra, vagina, and anus. Women who do these exercises report that they are more aware of their vagina, have more sensation in their pelvic area, and find sex more pleasurable. They also notice less leaking of urine when they cough, sneeze, or laugh, a very common symptom following menopause.

Dr. Kegel's exercises are simple and easy to do. They can be done anywhere—sitting, standing, or lying down. You may want to perform these exercises at least five times a day. They have been reported to help decrease symptoms of urinary incontinence in more than 50 percent of women who practice them. They can be performed as follows:

- Draw up the vaginal muscles slowly, hold for three seconds, then relax. Repeat the process ten times.

- Then tense and relax your vaginal muscles rapidly. Repeat the process ten times.

The Kegel exercises should be performed as part of a preventive program for vaginal and bladder health for the rest of your life along with any other therapy such as the use of estrogen.

Psychological Symptoms and Insomnia

Menopause can cause significant symptoms of emotional distress such as anxiety, irritability, mood swings, and depression as well as poor sleep quality. Regular aerobic exercise improves menopause-related emotional symptoms by improving the physiology and chemistry of the brain. This promotes healthy brain function and emotional well-being. After exercising, you will feel peaceful, calmer and even happier. You will even feel more refreshed and energized. How does exercise promote such significant emotional changes? Exercise brings better oxygenation and circulation to the brain and nerves. By opening up and dilating blood vessels of the head and brain, more nutrients flow to and waste products are removed from this vital system. In fact, 20 percent of the blood flow from the heart goes directly to the brain. The brain also utilizes a large share (about 20 percent) of the body's nutrients and energy.

Research studies of adults who exercise compared with similar adults who are sedentary show striking differences in a variety of mental functions. Adults engaged in an active exercise program have better concentration, clearer and quicker thinking, and better problem solving capabilities. After undertaking a regular exercise program, reaction time and short-term memory improved. This can be an important preventive benefit for women past midlife who want to preserve peak intellectual and mental capacity for the rest of their lives.

Not only does regular exercise induce functional improvements in the brain, it alters brain chemistry through the increased production of beta endorphins. Beta endorphins, chemicals released from the pituitary glands, act as natural opiates produced by the body. They are chemically similar to the pain reliever morphine but are two hundred times more potent. Endorphins have a dramatic effect on mood. When levels in the body are high, they improve a woman's general sense of well being.

Research studies demonstrate that brisk aerobic exercise such as running can increase beta endorphin levels as much as five-fold. Measurements taken a half hour after the end of an exercise session showed that beta endorphin levels were still higher than starting levels. Beta endorphins are thought to be responsible for the "runner's high" that marathon runners experience. Some women who exercise regularly report feelings of elation, euphoria, and even bliss.

Because beta endorphins elevate mood and promote well-being, exercise can also be an effective antidote for depression. While the standard treatment for depression is psychotherapy and antidepressant medication, a number of interesting chemical studies have shown that exercise helps relieve moderate depression in a significant fashion. This can be true in women of all ages, benefiting young women as well as women in their menopause years. One interesting study, done at the University of Virginia, studied depressed college students. During the study period, students who jogged regularly showed significant reduction in depression symptoms, while those students who did not exercise had virtually no change in their symptoms. This finding has significance for menopausal women when emotional symptoms of anxiety coexist with depression. Menopausal women often complain that their moods vacillate; for these women, exercise can be a powerful antidote, balancing and calming emotional upsets of all types.

Menopausal women often have difficulty sleeping at night. While hot flashes may initially awaken women in the middle of the night, falling back to sleep may be difficult. Some women find that once they are awake, their mind becomes active and may stay busy with "chatter" and self-talk for two to three hours.

Some women try strong sleeping medications or alcoholic beverages to induce sleep. In extreme cases, this can lead to drug and alcohol abuse as women increase their intake in an effort to sleep so they are not constantly exhausted from sleep deprivation during the day.

Exercise can also reduce insomnia by working off nervous energy and diffusing the fight-or-flight response to stress. After exercise, both the body and mind are calmer with the physiological parameters such as breathing and heart rate returning to a more healthful resting level. Regular exercise may also contribute to reducing alcohol and drug dependence. However, brisk exercise should not be done late in the day by women suffering from menopause-related insomnia because the energizing effects of the exercise are not desirable late at night. It is better to exercise earlier in the day if sleep induction is one of your main goals.

In summary, vigorous exercise brings blood to the brain as well as the endocrine glands and female reproductive tract. It can have a tremendously beneficial effect on mood, balancing and calming the emotions by helping promote healthier brain and nerve function. Anxiety, depression, and insomnia can be combated by a regular exercise program.

Osteoporosis

One of the most important reasons for engaging in regular physical activity during menopause is the prevention of osteoporosis. While the use of estrogen and nutrients, such as calcium and vitamin D, are necessary for building healthy bones and preventing loss of bone mass, they are not enough by themselves to prevent osteoporosis if a woman neglects physical activity and lives a sedentary life.

Bones demand exercise for their healthy maintenance. Lack of exercise will cause bone and muscle mass loss. This is true even in otherwise healthy, low-risk groups. For example, young people who are confined to bed for an illness lose bone mass.

While all aerobic exercise will strengthen your cardiovascular system and keeps your muscles fit and tuned, it will not necessarily preserve bone mass. To prevent osteoporosis, exercise must focus on the long bones of the body and make them work against the force of gravity. As a result, walking, trampolining, and dancing are excellent osteoporosis prevention exercises for the lower body. For the upper body, racket sports, weight lifting (with light weights), and tennis all help prevent bone loss in the torso and arms. An added benefit from participating in these activities is an increase in muscle mass and strength. In contrast, swimming will not help to preserve bone mass because water neutralizes the effect of gravity on the body. (Water activities, however, are excellent for women with muscular and joint problems, because they enhance flexibility and reduce stiffness.)

For best results, weight-bearing exercise must be practiced on a regular basis and in a sustained fashion. At least 30 minutes per session, three times a week should be done for bone protection. In fact, one study in *The New England Journal of Medicine* in 1991 reported that women who exercised three times a week and used calcium supplements lost significantly less bone mass (about one percent) over a two-year time period. However, women in the same study who did more than the recommended amount of exercise (the equivalent of two hours per day of brisk walking), lost no bone mass at all.

Unfortunately, many women over the ages of 45 to 50 are too inactive for adequate osteoporosis prevention. Many women have desk jobs requiring them to sit all day and there is little time to exercise. Other women choose not to exercise because they are self-conscious about their body shape or weight (which becomes more difficult to maintain with increasing age) or because their energy levels are diminished. In all of these cases, it is important to resist the urge to be sedentary. Keep moving and institute a regular exercise program combining both weight bearing and aerobic conditioning. Even short sessions of activity can make a difference.

Heart Disease

Heart disease is the biggest killer of women in the postmenopausal years; the incidence of heart disease increases ten fold in women between the ages of 55 and 65. Statistics such as these are unnecessary because heart disease can be prevented. The actual risk of developing heart disease, even if it is prevalent in your family, can be greatly lowered by practicing a healthy lifestyle. Reducing fat intake and emotional stress along with a regular program of aerobic exercise are important components of an effective heart disease prevention program.

Aerobic Exercise Benefits the Heart

Exercise conditions the heart and lungs to work more efficiently. A healthy heart is a well-functioning pump. It beats slowly and forcefully, circulating blood throughout the body with each stroke. Once an exercise program is initiated, the resting heart rate slows down quite rapidly. Research studies show that the beneficial changes can occur quickly, often within several months.

A healthier heart also reacts less dramatically during periods of stress. When nervous tension causes the adrenal glands to pump out stressor hormones, a conditioned heart will not experience a significant rise in heart rate. In a stressful situation, a fit person may have only a slight rise in heart rate, while a sedentary person may experience a terrifying pounding of the heart and shortness of breath. Not only does a fit person tend to stay calm and more in control of emotions during a difficult situation, but in periods of extreme stress, good physical conditioning may help prevent a heart attack.

Lungs function more efficiently with exercise, too. They expand more fully and fill with oxygen. Exercise helps dilate and expand the network of blood vessels in the body, so more blood reaches the muscles and vital organ systems. The effects of exercise will help prevent blood clotting and lower the level of fat in the blood vessels. A healthy heart and lungs mean greater endurance and physical energy. You can go through your daily activities more easily, with a sense of vigor and well-being.

Women who have been sedentary for a long period of time should not suddenly begin a vigorous program of aerobic activity. Starting a cardiovascular fitness program should be done gradually, and before beginning, I strongly recommend that you see your physician for a cardiovascular risk assessment. This is particularly important if you have a previous history of cardiovascular disease, diabetes mellitus, or high blood pressure. Your physician can identify any potential problems and help you tailor your exercise program.

Weight Control and Appearance

Exercise is an absolute necessity for most menopausal women for weight control and body tone. As our endocrine glands change with age, we tend to digest and metabolize food less efficiently. Pounds accumulate rapidly after menopause, as our bodies need fewer calories for maintenance. Some of my patients complained that they gained 10 to 15 pounds after menopause. These pounds can be very difficult to lose no matter how hard they diet. Many women eat smaller and smaller meals to maintain their weight. Older women who want to maintain their appearance are often in a state of chronic dieting to prevent "middle-age spread."

Luckily, exercise can provide midlife women with an antidote to unwanted pounds. Rather than cutting down caloric intake to starvation levels, increase your level of physical activity. Exercise allows you to maintain your weight far more easily than dieting because it burns calories and stimulates your metabolism. A regular aerobic program of walking, dancing, swimming, or other activity is a must to control your weight and allow you to look and feel your best. A regular exercise program also aids your appearance by helping preserve attractive body contours, toning muscles and improving skin condition. Exercise increases blood circulation to the skin, keeping the skin pink, soft, and supple. The skin of women who don't exercise frequently looks pale and unhealthy.

It is important, however, not to try to be too thin with the onset of menopause. Women who are too thin have lower estrogen levels and are at higher risk for such menopause problems as osteoporosis and hot flashes. Aim for a weight level and appearance that is attractive and not extreme—neither too thin nor obese. Set your weight and exercise program at a level that feels comfortable, is easy to maintain, and looks good.

Building a Personal Exercise Program

Evaluating your Fitness Level

As you move from a sedentary lifestyle to a regular exercise program, evaluate your level of fitness. It is important to know if you have any undiagnosed medical problems that could impact your proper level of activity. This includes problems such as thyroid disease, hypertension, and blood sugar imbalances commonly found in menopausal women. A complete medical examination is important for a menopausal woman beginning an exercise program after a long period of being sedentary.

Your physician should check your heart, lungs, pulse rate, and other physical parameters to evaluate your exercise fitness. In addition, blood and urine tests are frequently ordered. These tests can vary, based on the particular symptoms you report to your physician as well as the examination itself.

Depending on your age and symptoms, a general chemistry panel that checks the blood levels of minerals, as well as the health of various organs such as the thyroid may be required. If you don't understand any terms or tests your physician uses, ask for more information. An informed and educated woman can do a much better job in planning and participating in her own wellness program. Once you have received a clean bill of health or understand any health limitations, you are ready to begin planning your exercise program.

Choosing an Exercise Program

The type of exercise regimen you choose can vary greatly depending on the goals you wish to accomplish. If your main goal is to relieve menopause-related anxiety and stress and improve your general health and well-being, then aerobic exercise is best. This is because aerobic exercise promotes cardiovascular and respiratory health which, in turn, promotes relaxation and reduces the tendency toward menopause-related insomnia. Because it requires active work on the part of your skeletal and heart muscles, it reduces the muscle tension that often accompanies menopause-related nervous tension. Aerobic exercise includes jogging, walking, bicycle riding, skiing, swimming, dancing, jumping rope, and skating.

Women who are at high risk of osteoporosis will want to emphasize exercises that require weight-bearing stress on the long bones. Combining brisk walking with weight lifting or racquet sports can give the bones the workout they need and increase bone mass.

Women for whom sexuality is an important part of their emotional and physical well-being may find engaging in frequent sexual activity, or even massage, a pleasurable form of physical activity. For women who cannot participate in vigorous physical activity due to a pre-existing cardiovascular condition (or lack of energy), then slower-paced activities such as golf or walking could provide a helpful degree of physical exercise as well as the benefits of socializing.

Many menopausal women notice the onset of arthritis symptoms or muscle tightness and tension during this time. As an antidote, I recommend exercises such as yoga that promote joint and muscle flexibility. Yoga stretches are performed slowly along with deep breathing in a relaxed and careful manner. They are helpful in slowing down an anxious system whose physiology is set on overdrive.

Finally, gardening can promote peace of mind and relaxation along with physical activity. Pulling weeds and digging up the ground involve bending, lifting, and upper-body movements which rapidly dissipate anxiety.

Often, women may combine two or three types of exercise activities to meet a variety of goals. Whatever form of exercise you choose, make sure it meets the goals of promoting optimal health and well-being as well as providing abundant levels of energy.

Motivating Yourself to Exercise

If you encounter mental obstacles to beginning and sticking with a regular menopause exercise program, there are many ways to overcome this resistance. Be sure you are clear why you don't want to exercise so you can address the issues directly. Keeping the exercise diary found in the workbook section should help you pinpoint areas of resistance.

- Exercise at the time of day that feels most natural. For example, if you are a late riser, don't try to exercise early in the morning. Exercise when you are the least hurried and stressed by your schedule. If your longest amount of free time is in the late afternoon between work and dinner, put aside that time to engage in physical activity.

- Exercise in an attractive setting. If you run or walk, pick a setting near you that promotes peace and calm. Walk or run in a park, on a beach, or on a quiet residential street. Avoid areas with lots of cars and traffic congestion.

- Exercise with a friend or support person. This can be a great help in motivating and encouraging you to begin and stick with an exercise program.

- Use your mind to disconnect from your daily activities. Positive mental exercises can help you relax before starting physical activity. Many women find that a few minutes of doing visualizations (seeing themselves performing and enjoying the exercise routine in their minds) or saying affirmations (making positive statements about the benefits of exercise) prepares them for their exercise routine.

- Listen to music while you exercise. Many women find that the exercise period goes by more quickly and the process is more fun and enjoyable while listening to music. Be sure to choose music that is soft and relaxing if you are doing slow paced yoga or stretching exercises. This type of music will help improve your mood and relax you further. Fast paced music is more appropriate for quick-moving sessions of aerobic exercise.

- Be sure to choose an exercise activity that you enjoy. Don't pick an activity that you find boring. Refer to the Activity Chart at the end of this chapter if you need help in selecting an activity that looks interesting.

Beginning an Exercise Program for Menopause

Before you begin a menopause-relief exercise program, read the following guidelines. They will help you perform your exercise in an optimally beneficial manner. These guidelines are particularly useful for women just beginning regular exercise after leading a sedentary lifestyle. Getting a good start when beginning the program can make a major difference in how well you enjoy and stick to your chosen physical activity.

- During the first week or two of your program, build up your exercise level gradually. Keep initial exercise workouts short.

For example, you might start out exercising every other day for ten minutes. Increase the length of your sessions by five-minute increments until you are exercising between 30 and 60 minutes per session.

- Exercise in a relaxed and unhurried manner. Set aside adequate time so you do not feel rushed. Anytime you feel anxiety, panic, or excessive muscle tension, stop the exercise. Then, reevaluate your pace to see if it is too vigorous. Initially you might want to exercise with another person who can provide support and companionship.

- Wear loose, comfortable clothing. If you are doing stretching or yoga, work without socks to give your feet complete freedom of movement and to prevent slipping.

- Evacuate your bowels and/or bladder before you begin to exercise. Try to exercise at least 90 minutes before a meal and wait at least two hours after eating to exercise. Working out before dinner is particularly good because it helps diffuse tension that has accumulated throughout the day.

- Avoid exercising when ill or extremely stressed. Instead, do the stress-reduction exercises provided in this book.

- Move slowly and carefully when starting each exercise session. This promotes muscle flexibility and helps prevent injury.

- Breathe deeply and evenly when you are exercising; this will give you more endurance and you will tire less easily.

- Always rest for a few minutes after completing the exercises.

Activities for Menopausal Women

- walking
- bicycle riding
- skiing
- swimming
- aerobic dancing
- low-impact aerobics
- ice skating
- roller skating
- tennis
- ping-pong
- golf
- croquet
- bowling
- yoga
- stretching
- weight lifting
- gardening

Benefits of Exercise

- Helps relieve hot flashes
- Helps relieve vaginal and bladder atrophy
- Relieves anxiety, irritability, insomnia and depression
- Helps prevent osteoporosis
- Conditions heart, lungs, and muscles
- Helps prevent heart disease
- Helps control weight and improve appearance
- Improves function of vital organs such as digestive tract and nervous system
- Improves strength, stamina and flexibility
- Increases vigor and energy

16

Yoga for Menopause

*Y*oga stretches can benefit both the body and the mind, bringing energy and balance. This is particularly helpful to women who are currently in menopause or in menopause transition because their hormonal levels and body chemistry may be fluctuating rapidly. This can leave women feeling out-of-balance and truly victims of their changing bodies. Yoga exercises level out this physiological instability by relaxing and gently stretching every muscle in the body, promoting better blood circulation and oxygenation to all cells and tissues. This helps optimize the function of the endocrine glands and the organs of the female reproductive tract. Yoga exercises also improve the health and well-being of the digestive tract, nervous system, and all other organ systems.

The yoga exercises included in this chapter address many specific menopause-related symptoms and issues, such as bone strength, cardiovascular and breast health, of concern to all women past midlife. You may want to begin by trying all the stretches, then practicing on a regular basis those exercises that bring you the most symptom relief and general health benefits. If you prefer, begin with the exercises that offer relief for the specific symptoms of greatest concern.

General Techniques for Yoga

When doing yoga exercises, it is important that you focus and concentrate on the positions. First, let your mind visualize how the exercise is to look, and then follow with the correct body placement in the pose. The exercises are done through slow, controlled stretching movements. This slowness allows you to have greater control over your body movements. You minimize the possibility of injury and maximize the benefit to the particular area of the body where your attention is being focused.

Pay close attention to the initial instructions. Look at the placement of the body in the photographs. This is very important, for if the pose is practiced properly, you are much more likely to have relief from your symptoms.

In summary, as you begin these exercises:

- Visualize the pose in your mind, then follow with proper placement of the body.

- Move slowly through the pose. This will help promote flexibility of the muscles and prevent injury.

- Follow the breathing instructions provided in the exercise. Most important, do not hold your breath. Allow your breath to flow in and out easily and effortlessly.

Practicing yoga stretches regularly in a slow, unhurried fashion will gradually loosen your muscles, ligaments and joints. You may be surprised at how supple you can become over time. If you experience any pain or discomfort, you have probably overreached your current ability and should immediately reduce the amount of the stretching until you can proceed without discomfort. Be careful, as muscular injuries take time to heal. If you do strain a muscle, immediately apply ice to the injured area for ten minutes. Use the ice pack two to three times a day for several days. If the pain persists, see your doctor.

If you wish more background and information on yoga, refer to the books listed in the bibliography at the end of this book.

Stretch 1: The Locust

This exercise energizes the entire female reproductive tract, thyroid, liver, intestines and kidneys. It is helpful for premenopausal women with dysfunctional bleeding, as well as women with menopausal symptoms such as hot flashes because it improves circulation and oxygenation to the pelvic region, thereby promoting healthier ovarian function. This exercise also strengthens the lower back, abdomen, buttocks, and legs, and prevents lower back pain and cramps.

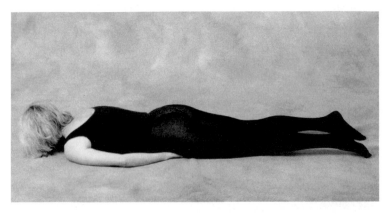

- Lie face down on the floor. Make fists with both your hands and place them under your hips. This prevents compression of the lumbar spine while doing the exercise.

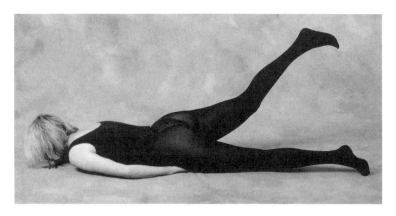

- Straighten your body and raise your right leg with an upward thrust as high as you can, keeping your hips on your fists. Hold for 5 to 20 seconds if possible.

- Lower the leg and slowly return to your original position. Repeat on the left side. Remember to keep your hips resting on your fists. Repeat 10 times.

- Repeat 10 times with both legs together.

Stretch 2: The Pump

This exercise improves blood circulation through the pelvis, thereby promoting healthier ovarian function. It helps relieve menopausal symptoms such as hot flashes and controls excessive bleeding in premenopausal women. The exercise helps calm anxiety and also strengthens the back and abdominal muscles.

- Lie down and press the small of your back into the floor. This permits you to use your abdominal muscles without straining your lower back.

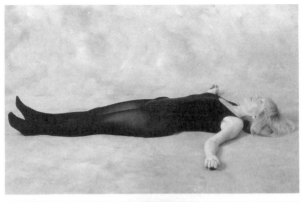

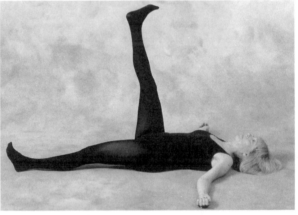

- Raise your right leg slowly while breathing in. Keep your back flat on the floor and let the rest of your body remain relaxed. Move your leg very slowly; imagine your leg being pulled up smoothly by a spring. Do not move your leg in a jerky manner. Hold for a few breaths. Lower your leg and breathe out.

- Repeat the same exercise on your left side. Then alternate legs, repeating the exercise 5 to 10 times.

Stretch 3: Wide-Angle Pose

This exercise opens the entire pelvic region and energizes the female reproductive tract, improving ovarian function as well as normalizing excessive or irregular menstrual flow; diminution of menopausal symptoms may also occur. It is helpful for varicose veins and improves circulation in the legs.

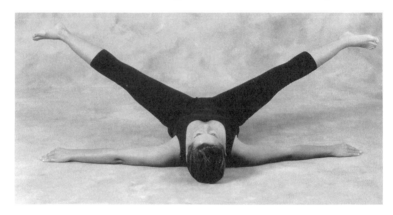

- Lie on your back with your legs against the wall and extended out in a V or an arc, and your arms extended to the side.

- Hips should be as close to the wall as possible, buttocks on the floor. Legs should be spread apart as far as they can and still remain comfortable. Breathing easily, hold for 1 minute, allowing the inner thighs to relax.

- Bring legs together and hold for 1 minute.

Stretch 4: Spinal Flex

This exercise energizes and rejuvenates the female reproductive tract and tones the abdominal organs (pancreas, liver and adrenals). It emphasizes freer pelvic movement with controlled breathing.

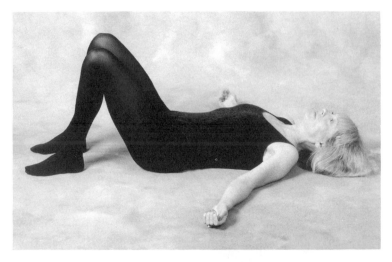

- Lie on your back with your knees bent and your feet on the floor close to your buttocks.

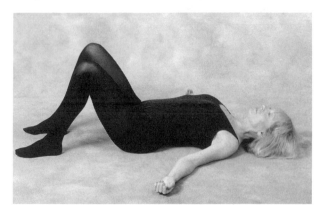

- Exhale and press the lower back into the floor, raising the buttocks slightly.

- Arch your back slightly.

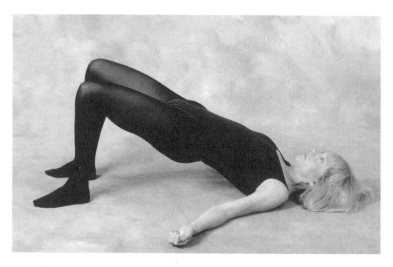

- Inhale and lift your lower back off the floor. This stretches the region from the sternum to the pelvis.

- Repeat this exercise 10 times. Always lift your navel up on the in-breath. Always elongate your spine and press the lower back down on the out-breath.

Stretch 5: Pelvic Arch

This is an excellent exercise for stretching the abdominal and pelvic muscles. Menopause-related vaginal and bladder symptoms are reduced by promoting better circulation and relaxation in the pelvic region. It is also helpful in reducing pelvic congestion.

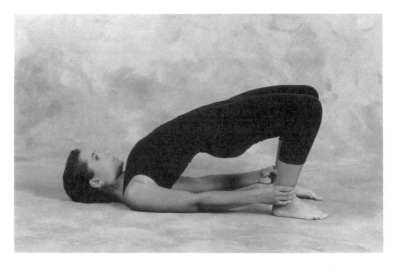

- Lie on your back with your knees bent. Spread your feet apart, flat on the floor.

- Place your hands around your ankles, holding them firmly.

- As you inhale, arch your pelvis up and hold for a few seconds. As you exhale, relax and lower your pelvis several times.

- Repeat this exercise several times.

Stretch 6: The Bow

This exercise helps relieve menopause-related fatigue and lack of vitality, elevating your mood and improving stamina. The exercise also stretches the entire spine and helps relieve lower back pain and cramps. It stretches the abdominal muscles and strengthens the back, hips and thighs. It also stimulates the digestive organs and endocrine glands.

- Lie face down on the floor, arms at your sides.

- Slowly bend your legs at the knees and bring your feet up toward your buttocks.

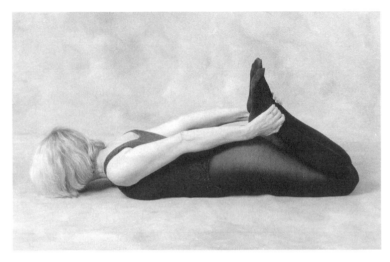

- Reach back with your arms and carefully take hold of first one foot and then the other. Flex your feet to make grasping them easier.

- Inhale and raise your trunk from the floor as far as possible and lift your head. Bring your knees as close together as possible.

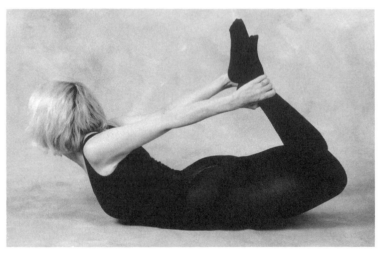

- Squeeze the buttocks while raising them off the floor. Imagine your body looking like a gently curved bow. Hold for 10 to 15 seconds.

- Slowly release the posture. Allow your chin to touch the floor and finally release your feet and return them slowly to the floor. Return to your original position. Repeat 5 times.

Stretch 7: Child's Pose

Excellent for calming anxiety and stress due to emotional causes, this exercise will also relieve menopause-related anxiety and irritability. The exercise gently stretches the lower back and is one of the most effective exercises for relieving menstrual cramps and low back pain.

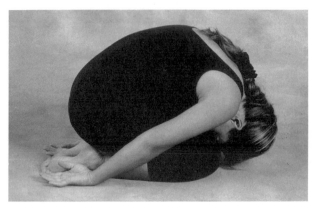

- Sit on your heels. Bring your forehead to the floor, stretching the spine as far over your head as possible.

- Close your eyes.

- Hold for as long as comfortable.

Stretch 8: The Sponge

This exercise relieves anxiety and stress due to emotional causes or menopause-related anxiety and tension. It relieves menstrual cramps and low back pain as well as reducing eye tension and swelling in the face.

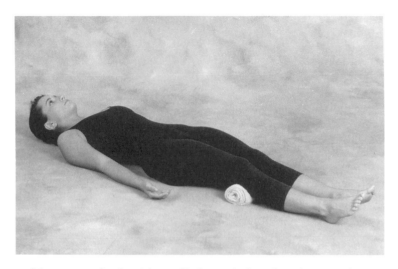

- Lie on your back with a rolled towel placed under your knees. Your arms should be at your sides, palms up.

- Close your eyes and relax your whole body. Inhale slowly, breathing from the diaphragm. As you inhale, visualize the energy in the air around you being dawn in through your entire body. Imagine your body is porous and open like a sponge, drawing in this energy and revitalizing every cell of your body.

- Exhale slowly and deeply, allowing all tension to drain from your body.

Stretch 9: Dollar Pose

This pose reduces anxiety and nervous tension and will help eliminate tension headaches and insomnia. It improves flexibility of the spine, reducing stiffness and back pain.

- Lie on your back with your legs bent and your feet together. Place your hands on the sides of both ankles to keep your legs together.

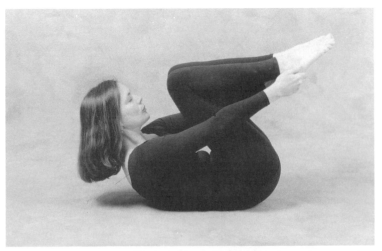

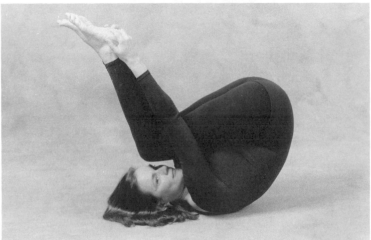

- As you inhale, raise your legs up over your head. Make sure that the posture is comfortable by adjusting the angle of your legs. To do this, bend your knees to apply pressure between the shoulder blades.

- Hold this posture for one minute, breathing slowly and deeply.

- Return to the original position, lying flat on your back with your eyes closed. Relax in this position for several minutes.

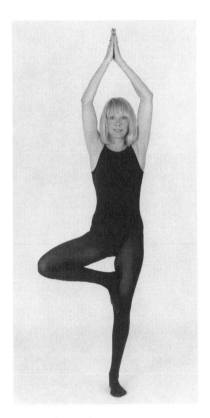

Stretch 10: Tree

If your goal is to strengthen bone mass by increasing weight bearing on the legs, hips and spine, this exercise will help you accomplish increasing bone mass. It also improves balance and posture.

- Standing erect, focus your eyes on a stationary point. Place one foot against the opposite thigh, so that one leg is bearing your weight.

- Slowly raise your arms over your head. Hold for a count of 5.

   Reverse sides.

   Repeat 3 times.

Note: You may place one hand on the wall for support if needed.

Stretch 11: Chest Expander

This exercise increases circulation to the upper half of the body, energizing and stimulating the body. It also loosens and stretches tense muscles in the upper body, especially the shoulder and back, and expands the lungs.

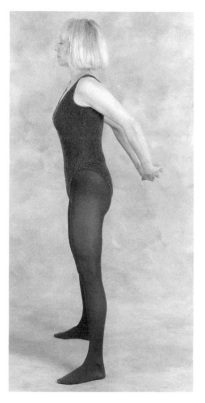

- Stand easily. Arms should be at your sides; feet are hip distance apart.

- Extend your arms forward until your palms touch.

- Bring your arms slowly and gracefully back until you can clasp them behind your back.

- Exhale, then straighten your clasped hands and arms as far as you can without discomfort. Remember to stand upright; body should not bend forward. Breathe deeply into chest.

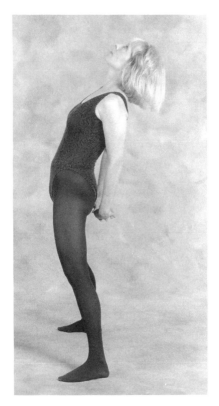

- Inhale deeply and bend backward from the waist. Keep your hands clasped and your arms held high.

- Drop your head backward a few inches and look upward as you relax your shoulders and the back of your neck.

- Hold this position for a few seconds.

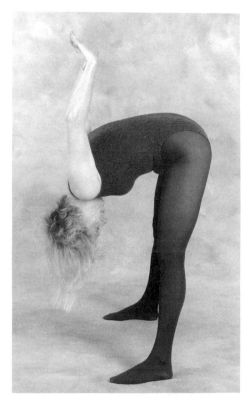

- As you hold your breath, bend forward at the waist, bringing your clasped hands and arms up over your back.

- Relax your neck muscles and keep your knees straight.

- Hold for a few seconds.

- Exhale as you return to the upright position. Unclasp your hands and allow your arms to rest easily at your sides.

- Repeat entire sequence 3 times.

Choosing the Right Yoga Technique

From among the many specific yoga poses in this chapter, you can choose the best exercises to provide relief for your personal menopausal symptoms by using the accompanying chart. Try all the poses that pertain to your specific symptoms to see which ones bring you the most relief and practice those poses on a regular basis along with your exercise program. The combination of yoga stretches plus a good aerobic and strength-building program should help relieve and delay menopause-related symptoms and improve your general state of health.

Symptoms	*Exercise*
Entire female reproductive tract	Locust, Pump, Wide-Angle Pose, Spinal Flex, Pelvic Arch, Bow
Excessive or irregular menstrual bleeding	Locust, Pump, Wide-Angle Pose
Hot flashes	Locust, Pump, Wide-Angle Pose, Spinal Flex, Pelvic Arch, Bow
Insomnia	Child's Pose, Sponge, Dollar Pose
Psychological symptoms— anxiety, depression, fatigue	Bow, Child's Pose, Sponge, Dollar Pose
Vaginal atrophy and bladder symptoms	Locust, Pump, Wide-Angle Pose, Spinal Flex, Pelvic Arch, Bow
Osteoporosis	Tree
Cardiovascular health	Chest Expander
Breast health	Chest Expander

17

Acupressure for Menopause

*A*cupressure is a traditional Oriental healing technique of applying finger pressure to specific points on the body to help treat and prevent symptoms of various ailments. Over the years, many of my menopause patients have tried acupressure and it really works! Acupuncture, where the points are stimulated by needles, is done by a trained professional. While acupressure is not a cure-all, many women have reported significant relief from such common menopausal symptoms as hot flashes, fatigue, insomnia and mood swings.

How Does Acupressure Work?

When specific acupressure points are pressed, they create changes on two levels. On the physical level, acupressure affects muscular tension, blood circulation, and other physiological parameters. On a more subtle level, traditional Oriental healing believes that acupressure also builds the body's life energy to promote healing. Acupressure is based on the belief of a life energy in the body called *chi*. It is different from, yet similar to, electromagnetic energy. Health is a state in which the *chi* is present in sufficient amounts and is equally distributed throughout the body energizing all the cells and tissues of the body.

The life energy runs through the body in channels called meridians. When working in a healthy manner, these channels distribute the energy evenly throughout the body, sometimes on the surface of the skin and at times deep inside the body in the organs. Disease occurs when the energy flow in a meridian is blocked or stopped. As a result, the internal organs that correspond to the meridians can show symptoms of disease. The meridian flow can be corrected by stimulating the points on the skin surface. These points can be treated easily by acupressure. When the normal flow of energy through the body is resumed, the body can then heal itself spontaneously.

You or a friend can stimulate the acupressure points through safe and painless finger pressure by following simple instructions.

How to Perform Acupressure

Acupressure should be done when you are relaxed. The room should be warm and quiet. Make sure your hands are clean and nails trimmed (to avoid bruising). If your hands are cold, rinse them under warm water.

Work on the side of the body that has the most discomfort. If both sides are equally uncomfortable, choose either side. Just working on one side will relieve the symptoms on both sides. Energy or information seems to transfer from one side to the other.

Look carefully at the illustration for the exercise. Hold each point indicated in the exercise with a steady pressure for one to three minutes, applying pressure slowly with the tips or balls of the fingers. It is best to place several fingers over the area of the point. If you feel resistance or tension in the area where you are applying pressure, you may want to increase the pressure slightly. Make sure your hand is comfortable; if your hand starts to feel tense or tired, release the pressure a bit. The acupressure point may feel tender; this means the energy pathway or meridian is blocked.

During the treatment, the tenderness in the point should slowly fade. You may also have a sense of energy radiating from this point into the body. Many women describe this sensation as very pleasant. Don't worry if you don't feel it—not everyone does. The main goal is relief from your symptoms.

Breathe gently while doing each exercise. The photograph accompanying the exercise will help you visualize the point you will hold. All of these points correspond to specific points on the acupressure meridians. You may apply acupressure to the points once a day, or more if you continue to have symptoms.

Acupressure Exercises

Exercise 1: Balances the Entire Reproductive System

This exercise balances the energy of the female reproductive tract and is a useful exercise to begin your acupressure program. It also helps relieve low back pain and abdominal discomfort.

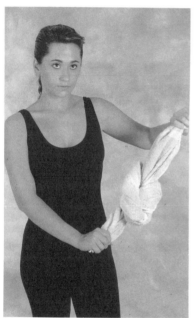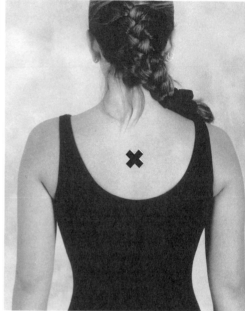

Equipment. This exercise uses a knotted hand towel to put pressure on hard-to-reach areas of the back. Place the knotted towel on these points while your hands are on other points. This increases your ability to unblock the energy pathways of your body.

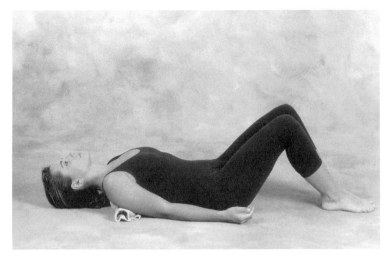

- Lie on the floor with your knees up. As you lie down, place the towel between the shoulder blades on your spine. Hold each step 1 to 3 minutes.

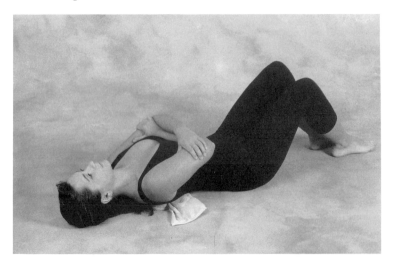

- Cross your arms on your chest. Press your thumbs against the right and left inside upper arms.

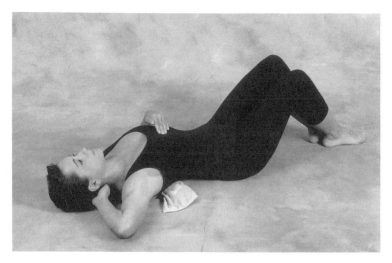

- Left hand holds point at the base of the sternum (breastbone). Right hand holds point at the base of the head (at the junction of the spine and the skull).

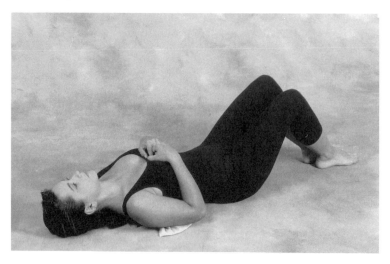

- Interlace your fingers. Place them below your breasts. Fingertips should press directly against the body.

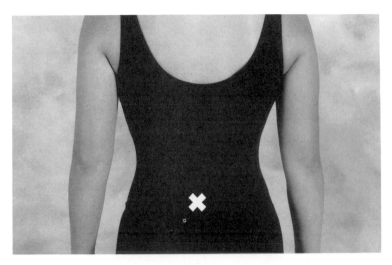

- Move the knotted towel along the spine to the waistline.

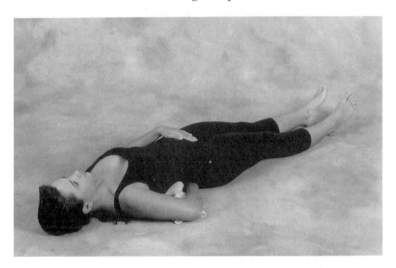

- Left hand should be placed at the top of the pubic bone, pressing down. Right hand holds point on tailbone.

Exercise 2: Relieves Excessive Menstrual Bleeding

This sequence balances the points on the spleen meridian. It is useful in controlling excessive menstrual bleeding, a common problem of premenopausal women. It also helps relieve premenstrual bloating and fluid retention and minimizes weight gain in the period leading up to menstruation which can be accentuated as women transition into menopause.

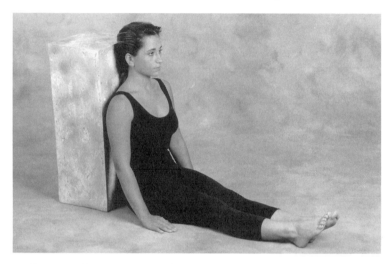

- Sit up and prop your back against a chair, or lie down and put your lower legs on a chair. Hold each step 1 to 3 minutes.

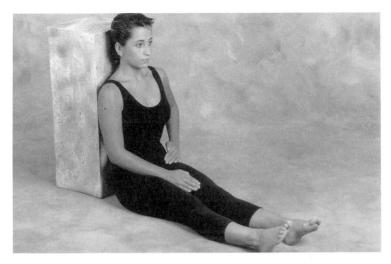

- Left hand is placed in the crease of the groin where you bend your leg, one-third to one-half way between the hip bone and the outside edge of the pubic bone. Right hand holds a spot 2 to 3 inches above the knee.

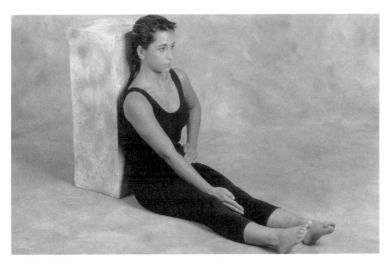

- Left hand remains in the crease of the groin.

  Right hand holds point below inner part of knee. To find the point, follow the curve of the bone just below the knee. Hold the underside of the curve with your fingers.

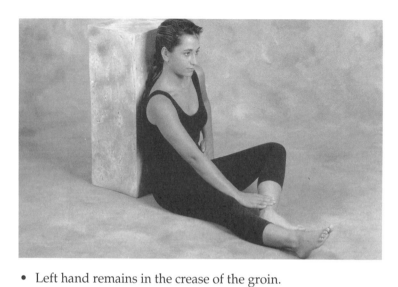

- Left hand remains in the crease of the groin.

  Right hand holds the inside of the shin. To find this point, go 4 fingerwidths above the ankle bone. The point is just above the top finger.

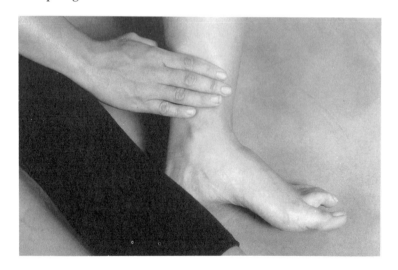

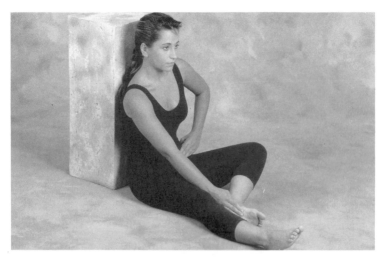

- Left hand remains in the crease of the groin.

  Right hand holds the edge of the instep. To find the point, follow the big toe bone up until you hit a knobby, prominent small bone.

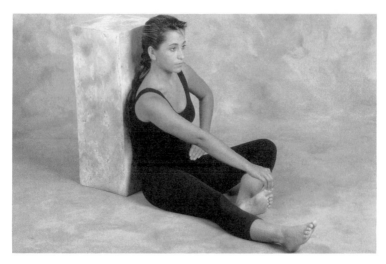

- Left hand remains in the crease of the groin.

  Right hand holds the big toe over the nail, front and back of the toe.

Exercise 3: Relieves Hot Flashes and Emotional Tension

This exercise helps relieve hot flashes by stimulating the entire endocrine system. It involves a very powerful point for the pituitary gland, the master regulator of the ovaries. This point also helps relax the emotional tension that many women feel during early menopause and relieves eye strain, headaches, and hay fever.

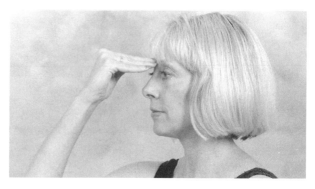

- Sit upright on a chair.

- Right hand holds point directly between the eyebrows, where the bridge of the nose meets the forehead. Hold the point for 1 to 3 minutes.

Exercise 4: Relieves Hot Flashes, Menopausal Fatigue, Anxiety, and Depression

This exercise helps relieve hot flashes as well as menopausal-related fatigue, insomnia, anxiety, and depression. The exercise will also relieve fatigue, anxiety, and depression women may experience prior to their menstrual periods.

- Sit up and prop your back against a chair. Hold each step 1 to 3 minutes.

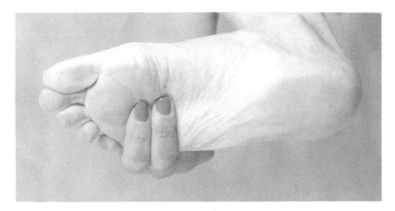

- Right hand holds point at the base of the ball of the right foot. This point is located between the two pads of the foot.

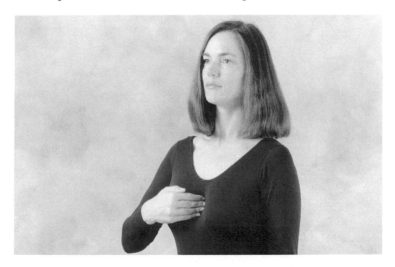

- Right hand holds point in the center of your breastbone, at the level of the heart. Your fingers will fit into the indentations in this bone.

Exercise 5: Relieves
Menopause-Related Insomnia

This exercise helps relieve insomnia and anxiety symptoms commonly seen in menopause. In Oriental medicine, these points are called "joyful sleep" and "calm sleep."

• Sit comfortably and hold these points for 1 to 3 minutes.

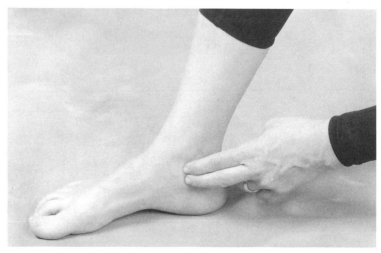

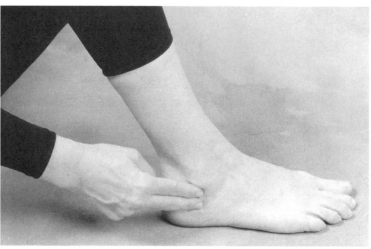

- Left hand holds point on the inside of the right anklebone. This point is located in the indentation directly below the inner ankle bone.

- Right hand holds point located in the indentation below the right outer ankle bone.

Repeat this exercise holding the points on the left foot.

Exercise 6: Relieves Vaginal and Urinary Tract Atrophy and Promotes Healthy Bones

This exercise helps relieve symptoms of vaginal dryness and insufficient vaginal lubrication seen in menopausal women with inadequate estrogen stimulation of the vaginal tissues. These points are also used to promote strong and healthy bones. The second step in this sequence helps promote bladder health during menopause.

- Sit on the floor with the knees bent or sit up and prop your back against a chair. Hold each step for 1 to 3 minutes.

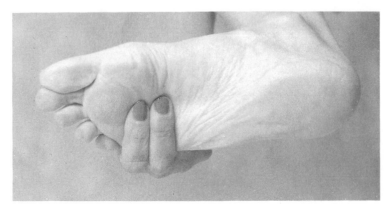

- Right hand holds point at the base of the ball of the right foot. The point is located between the two pads of the foot.

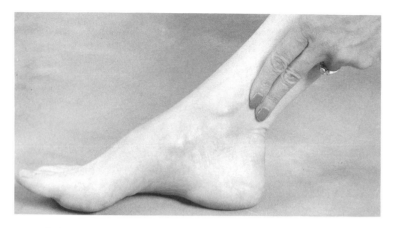

- Left hands holds the point midway between the inside of the right anklebone and the Achilles tendon. The Achilles tendon is located at the back of the ankle.

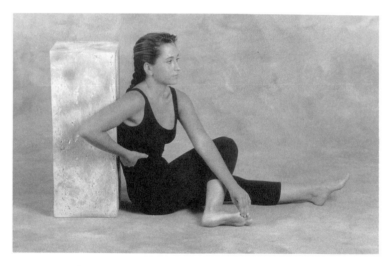

- Move left hand 1 inch above the waist on the muscle to the side of the spine. Right hand holds the point on the outside of the foot, just behind the little toe.

Exercise 7: Improves Cardiovascular Health

This exercise strengthens the cardiovascular system. Health problems involving this system are the major cause of death in postmenopausal women.

- Sit or stand in a comfortable position. Hold each step for 1 to 3 minutes.

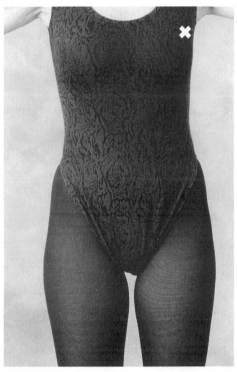

- Right hand holds point at the base of the armpit on the chest.

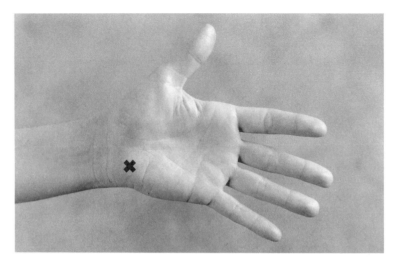

- Right hand holds point at base of left wrist below the little finger.

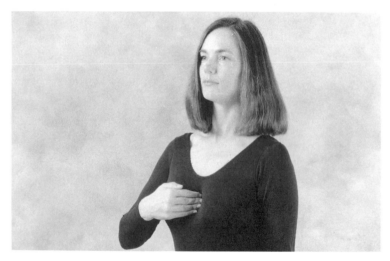

- Right hand holds point in the center of your breast bone, at the level of the heart. Your fingers will fit into the indentations in this bone.

Exercise 8: Improves Breast Health

This point improves breast health by stimulating the pituitary, the master gland that regulates the output of hormones affecting the health of the breast tissue.

- Sit upright in a chair or stand up. Hold each step for 1 to 3 minutes.

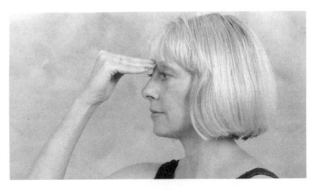

- Right hand holds point directly between the eyebrows where the bridge of the nose meets the forehead.

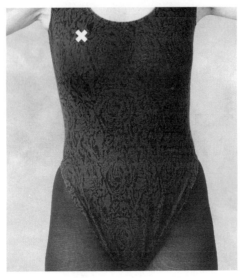

- Right hand holds point on right side of chest directly above the breast in line with the nipple . Point is between the third and fourth ribs.

Choosing the Right Exercises

You can use the chart to select acupressure exercises most useful for your specific symptoms. Initially, try all those that pertain to your symptoms. You may find that certain ones make you feel better than others. Practice the acupressure points that bring you the most relief.

Symptoms	Acupressure Exercise
Entire female reproductive tract	1
Excessive or irregular menstrual bleeding	2
Hot flashes	3, 4
Insomnia	4, 5
Psychological symptoms—anxiety, depression, fatigue	3, 4
Vaginal atrophy	6
Bladder symptoms	6
Osteoporosis	6
Cardiovascular health	7
Breast health	8

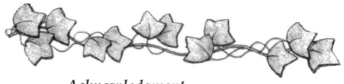

Acknowledgment

The author and publisher wish to extend a special acknowledgment to Shelly Reeves-Smith and Cracom Corporation for permission to reproduce the creative line drawings found in the food section of this book. These and additional drawings, together with a collection of wonderful recipes, may be found in the cookbook *Just a Matter of Thyme* available in your local gift or book store. Inquiries may be addressed to Among Friends, P.O. Box 1476, Camdenton, MO 65020 or call toll free (800) 377-3566.

Health & Lifestyle Resources

As a strong advocate for women, I am committed to providing the information and education they need for optimal health. The more access women have to information about their important health issues, the more they can participate in and promote their own well-being. Because so many women need these resources, I have made them available through *The LIFECYCLES Center for Women*. We currently stock the following items:

Books The Women's Health Series books are listed on the copyright page.

Foods
Flax Oil
Flax and Borage Oil Capsules

Vitamin and Mineral Supplements
PMS Nutritional System
Menopause Nutritional System
Woman's Daily Spectrum Nutritional System
Daily Iron Nutritional System
"Unwind," A Relaxant Formula
Women's Water Balance

Women's Personal Products Vitamin E Vaginal Suppositories to help soothe the vaginal tissues.

If you are interested in obtaining any of our self-help programs and resources for women, contact:

The LIFECYCLES Center
101 First Street, Suite 441
Los Altos, CA 94022-2706
(800) 862-9876 (For orders only)
FAX (415) 965-4311

Bibliography

Part I, Books

Barbach, L., PhD. *The Pause*. New York: Dutton Books, 1993.

Beard, M., M.D., and L. Curtis, M.D. *Menopause and The Years Ahead*. Tucson, AZ: Fisher Books, 1991.

Gaby, A. R., M.D. *Preventing and Reversing Osteoporosis: Every Woman's Essential Guide*. Rocklin, CA: Prima Publishing, 1994.

Gambrell, R. D., M.D. *Estrogen Replacement Therapy*. Dallas, TX: Essential Medical Information Systems, Inc., 1989.

Greenwood, S., M.D. *Menopause Naturally*. San Francisco, CA: Volcano Press, 1992.

Jacobowitz, R. *150 Most-Asked Questions About Menopause*. New York: Hearst Books, 1993.

Lee, J. R. *Natural Progesterone: The Multiple Roles of a Remarkable Hormone*. Sebastopol, CA: BLL Publishing, 1992.

Legato, M., M.D. *The Female Heart*. New York: Avon Books, 1991.

London, S., M.D., and H. T. Chihal, M.D. *Menopause Clinical Concepts*. Amityville, NY: Essential Medical Information Systems, Inc., 1989.

Nachtigall, L., M.D. *Estrogen*. New York: Harper Perennial, 1991.

Notolovitz, M., M.D., and D. Tonnessen. *Menopause and Midlife Health*. New York: St. Martin's Press, 1993.

Sheehy, G. *The Silent Passage*. New York: Simon & Schuster, 1993.

Utian, W., M.D., and R. Jacobowitz. *Managing Your Menopause*. New York: Fireside Books, 1990.

Part I, Articles

Alberecht, B. H., et al. Objective evidence that placebo and oral medroxyprogesterone acetate therapy diminish menopausal vasomotor flushes. *American Journal of Obstetrics and Gynecology*. 1981; 139:631–5.

Aloia, J. F., et al. Risk factors for postmenopausal osteoporosis. *American Journal of Medicine*. 1985; 78:95–100.

Avioli, L. V. Adjunctive modes of therapy for postmenopausal osteoporosis. *Postgraduate Medicine Special Report*. September 1987; 21–8.

Baber, R. J., and J. W. Studd. Hormone replacement therapy and cancer. *British Journal of Hospital Medicine*. February 1989; 41(2):142–9.

Bachmann, C. A., et al. Sexual repercussions of aging. *Contemporary OB/Gyn*. 1987; 29:1–72.

Barrett-Connor, E. Editorial: Postmenopausal estrogen replacement and breast cancer. *New England Journal of Medicine*. 1989; 321:319–20.

Barrett-Connor, E. Epidemiology and the menopause: A global overview. *International Journal Fertility Menopausal Study*. 1993; 1:6–14.

Barrett-Connor, E., and V. Miller. Estrogens, lipids, and heart disease. *Clinics in Geriatric Medicine.* February 1993; 9(1):57–67.

Beard, M. K., and L. R. Curtis. Libido, menopause and estrogen replacement therapy. *Postgraduate Medicine.* 1989; 86:1:225–8.

Bergkvist, L., et al. The risk of breast cancer after estrogen and estrogen-progestin replacement. *New England Journal of Medicine.* 1989; 321:293.

Brincat, M., et al. Long-term effects of the menopause and sex hormones on skin thickness. *British Journal of Obstetrics and Gynecology.* 1986; 92:256–9.

Brzezinski, A., et al. Editorial: Menopause and hormone replacement therapy in relation to atherosclerotic heart disease. *Harefuah.* April 1991; 120(7):419–21.

Burckhardt, P., and C. H. Michel. The peak bone mass concept. *Clinical Rheumatology.* 1989; 8:16.

Burkman, R. T., Jr. Strategies for reducing cardiovascular risk in women. *Journal of Reproductive Medicine.* March 1991; 36(3 Supplement):238–46.

Bush, T. L., et al. Estrogen use and all-cause mortality: Preliminary results from the lipid research clinics program follow-up study. *Journal of the American Medical Association.* 1983; 249:903–6.

Campbell, S. and M. Whitehead. Oestrogen therapy and the menopausal syndrome. *Clinical Obstetrics and Gynecology.* 1977; 4:31–47.

Chetkowski, R. J., et al. Biologic effects of transdermal estradiol. *New England Journal of Medicine.* 1986; 314:1615–20.

Christiansen, C., et al. Bone mass in postmenopausal women after withdrawal of oestrogen/gestagen replacement therapy. *Lancet.* 1981; 1:459–61.

Christiansen, J. J., et al. Cigarette smoking, serum estrogens and bone loss during hormone replacement early after menopause. *New England Journal of Medicine.* 1985; 313:973.

Colditz, C. A., et al. Menopause and the risk of coronary heart disease in women. *New England Journal of Medicine.* 1987; 316:1105–10.

Collins, J., et al. Estrogen use and survival in endometrial cancer. *Lancet.* 1980; 961–4.

Coulan, C. B. Age, estrogens and psyche. *Clinical Obstetrics & Gynecology.* March 1981; 24(1):219–29.

Cummings, S. R. Evaluating the benefits and risks of postmenopausal hormone therapy. *American Journal of Medicine.* November 1991; 91(5B):14S–18S.

Cummings, S. R., et al. Lifetime risks of hip, Colles', or vertebral fracture and coronary heart disease among white postmenopausal women. *Archives of Internal Medicine.* November 1989; 149(11):2445–8.

Dennerstein, L. Psychologic changes. *Menopause. Yearbook Medical Publishers* 1987; 115

Dupont, W. D., et al. Influence of exogenous estrogens, proliferative breast disease, and other variables on breast cancer risk. *Cancer.* 1989; 63:948–57.

Dupont, W. D., and D. L. Page. Menopausal estrogen replacement therapy and breast cancer. *Archives of Internal Medicine.* 1991; 151:67–72.

Eiken, P. A. Hormone replacement therapy and risk of ischemic heart disease and other causes of death. A review of studies published 1970–1992. Ugeskrift for Laeger. December 1993; 155(50):4067–76.

Erlik, Y., et al. Association of waking episodes with menopausal hot flushes. *Journal of the American Medical Association.* 1981; 245:1741–4.

Ettinger, B. Hormone replacement therapy and coronary heart disease. *Obstetrics and Gynecology Clinics of North America.* December 1990; 17(4):741–57.

Falkeborn, M., et al. Hormone replacement therapy and the risk of stroke. Follow-up of a population-based cohort in Sweden. *Archives of Internal Medicine.* May 1993; 153(10):1201–9.

Farish, E., et al. Lipoprotein and apolipoprotein levels in postmenopausal women on continuous oestrogen/progestogen therapy. *British Journal of Obstetrics and Gynecology.* 1989; 96:358–64.

Felson, D. T., et al. The effect of postmenopausal estrogen therapy on bone density in elderly women. *The New England Journal of Medicine.* October 1993; 329(16):1141–6.

Finucane, F. F., et al. Decreased risk of stroke among postmenopausal hormone users. Results from a national cohort. *Archives of Internal Medicine.* January 1993; 153(1):73–9.

Fletcher, C. D., et al. Short-term changes in lipoproteins and apoproteins during cyclical oestrogen-progestogen replacement therapy. *Maturitas.* December 1991; 14(1):33–42.

Flowers, C. E., et al. Mechanisms of uterine bleeding in postmenopausal patients receiving estrogen alone or with a progestin. *Obstetrics and Gynecology.* 1983; 61(2):135–43.

Gambrell, R. D., Jr., et al. Role of estrogens and progesterone in the etiology and prevention of endometrial cancer: A review. *American Journal of Obstetrics and Gynecology.* 1983; 146:696.

Gambrell, R. D., Jr., et al. Decreased incidence of breast cancer in postmenopausal estrogen-progestogen users. *Obstetrics and Gynecology.* 1983; 62:435.

Gangar, E. Appropriate use of HRT postmenopause. *Nursing Standard.* November 1992; 7(9):28–30.

Gibbons, W. E., et al. Biochemical and histologic effects of sequential estrogen/progestin therapy on the endometrium of postmenopausal women. *American Journal of Obstetrics and Gynecology.* 1986; 154:456–61.

Gold, E. B. Smoking and the menopause. *Menopause Management.* November 1990; 3(3):9–11.

Gordon, T., et al. Menopause and coronary heart disease: The Framingham study. *Annals of Internal Medicine.* 1978; 89:157–61.

Haarbo, J., et al. Serum lipids, lipoproteins, and apolipoproteins during postmenopausal estrogen replacement therapy combined with either 19-nortestosterone derivatives or 17-hydroxyprogesterone derivatives. *American Journal of Medicine.* 1991; 90:584–9.

Hammond, M. G. Managing menopausal signs and symptoms. *Drug Therapy.* December 1984; 154–23.

Hammond, C. B. Estrogen replacement therapy: What the future holds. *American Journal of Obstetrics and Gynecology.* 1989; 161:1864–8.

Hazzard, W. R. Estrogen replacement and cardiovascular disease, serum lipids and blood pressure effects. *American Journal of Obstetrics and Gynecology.* 1989; 161:1847–53.

Henderson, B. E., et al. Menopausal estrogen therapy and hip fractures. *Annals of Internal Medicine.* 1981; 95:28.

Henderson, B. E., et al. Estrogen use and cardiovascular disease. *American Journal of Obstetrics and Gynecology.* 1986; 154:1181–6.

Henderson, B. E., et al. Decreased mortality in users of estrogen replacement therapy. *Archives of Internal Medicine.* 1991; 151:75–8.

Hillard, T. C., et al. The long-term risks and benefits of hormone replacement therapy. *Journal of Clinical Pharmacy and Therapeutics.* August 1991; 16(4):231–45.

Jensen, J., et al. Cigarette smoking, serum estrogens and bone loss during hormone-replacement therapy early after menopause. *New England Journal of Medicine.* 1985; 313:973–5.

Jensen, J., et al. Cyclic changes in serum cholesterol and lipoproteins following different doses of combined postmenopausal hormone replacement therapy. *British Journal of Obstetrics and Gynecology.* 1986; 93:613–18.

Jensen, J., et al. Continuous estrogen-progesterone treatment and serum lipoproteins in postmenopausal women. *British Journal of Obstetrics and Gynecology.* 1987; 94:130–5.

Jensen, J., et al. Long-term effects percutaneous estrogens and oral progesterone on serum lipoproteins in postmenopausal women. *American Journal of Obstetrics and Gynecology.* 1987; 156:66–71.

Kable, W., et al. Lipid changes after hormone replacement therapy for menopause. *Journal of Reproductive Medicine.* May 1990; 35(5):512.

Kelsey, J. L., et al. Risk factors for hip fracture. *New England Journal of Medicine.* 1987; 316(4):173–7.

Kiel, D. P., et al. Smoking eliminates the protective effect of oral estrogens on the risk for hip fracture among women. *Annals of Internal Medicine.* 1992; 116:716–21.

Krauss, R. M. Lipids and lipoproteins in postmenopausal women. *Postgraduate Medicine Special Report.* September 1987; 56–60.

Laufer, L. R., et al. Estrogen replacement therapy by transdermal estradiol administration. *American Journal of Obstetrics and Gynecology* 1983; 146:533.

Laufer, L. R., et al. Effect of clonidine on hot flashes in postmenopausal women. *Obstetrics and Gynecology.* 1982; 60:583–6.

Leiblum, S., et al. Vaginal atrophy in the postmenopausal woman. *Journal of the American Medical Association.* 1983; 249:2195–7.

Lindenstrom, E., et al. Lifestyle factors and risk of cerebrovascular disease in women. The Copenhagen City Heart Study. *Stroke.* October 1993; 24(10):1468–72.

Lindsay, R., et al. The minimum effective dose of estrogen for prevention of postmenopausal bone loss. *Obstetrics and Gynecology.* 1984; 63:759–63.

Lindsay, R. Estrogen replacement for osteoporosis. *Current Trends in Estrogen Replacement Therapy.* 1986.

Lindsay, R. Identification of bone loss and its prevention by sex steroids. *Postgraduate Medicine. Special Report.* September 1987; 13–20.

Lobo, R. A., et al. Cardiovascular effects of estrogen deprivation. *Postgraduate Medicine. Special Report.* September 1987; 29–38.

Lobo, R. A. Cardiovascular implications of estrogen replacement therapy. *Obstetrics and Gynecology.* 1990; 185S–25S.

Lufkin, E. G. Estrogen efficacy and side effects in the prevention and treatment of osteoporosis. *Current Perspective on Managing the Premenopausal and Postmenopausal Woman.* December 8, 1990.

Lufkin, E. G., et al. Estrogen replacement therapy: Current recommendations. *Mayo Clinic Proceedings.* 1988; 27:201–23.

Lufkin, E. G., et al. Treatment of postmenopausal osteoporosis with transdermal estrogen. *Annals of Internal Medicine.* 1992; 117:1–9.

Mandel, F. P., et al. Effects of progestins on bone metabolism in postmenopausal women. *Journal of Reproductive Medicine.* 27(8):511–4.

Matthews, K. A., et al. Menopause and risk factors for coronary heart disease. *New England Journal of Medicine.* 1989; 321:641–6.

Mason, W. S., and J. T. Hargrove. Bioavailability of oral micronized progesterone. *Fertility and Sterility.* 1985; 44:622–6.

Meade, T. W., and A. Berra. Hormone replacement therapy and cardiovascular disease. *British Medical Bulletin.* April 1992; 48(2):276–308.

Meldrum, D. R., et al. Gonadotropins, estrogens, and adrenal steroids during menopausal hot flash. *Journal of Clinical Endocrinology and Metabolism.* 1980; 50:585–9.

Nabulsi, A. A., et al. Association of hormone-replacement therapy with various cardiovascular risk factors in postmenopausal women. *New England Journal of Medicine.* 1993; 328:1069–75.

Nachtigall, L. E. Estrogen replacement: Which postmenopausal women benefit? *Female Patient.* 1987; 12:72–86.

Nachtigall, L. E., et al. Evaluating the newly menopausal woman. *Contemporary OB/Gyn.* 1985; 25(5):68–92.

Nachtigall, L. E., and M. J. Nachtigall. Hormone replacement therapy. *Current Opinion in Obstetrics and Gynecology.* December 1992; 4(6):907–13.

Nagaman, M., et al. Treatment of menopausal hot flashes with transdermal administration of clonidine. *American Journal of Obstetrics and Gynecology.* 1987; 156:561–5.

Namburdiri, D. E., et al. Sexuality after menopause. *Female Patient.* 1987; 12:20–6.

Nordin, B. E. C., et al. A placebo-controlled trial of ethinyl estradiol and norethisterone to climateric women. *Maturitas.* 1980; 2:247–51.

Notelovitz, M., et al. Combination estrogen and progestogen replacement therapy does not adversely affect coagulation. *Obstetrics and Gynecology.* 1983; 62:596–600.

Notelovitz, M. Osteoporosis: A decade's findings in prevention, diagnosis and treatment. *Female Patient.* 1986; 11:49–60.

Ottosson, U. B., et al. Subfractions of high-density lipoprotein cholesterol during estrogen replacement therapy: A comparison between progestogens and natural progesterone. *American Journal of Obstetrics and Gynecology.* 1985; 151:746–50.

Padwick, M. L., et al. Efficacy, acceptability and metabolic effects of transdermal estradiol in the management of postmenopausal women. *American Journal of Obstetrics and Gynecology.* 1985; 152:1092–99.

Persson, I., et al. Risk of endometrial cancer after treatment with oestrogens alone or in conjunction with progestogens: Results of prospective study. *British Medical Journal.* 1989; 298:147–51.

Pfeffer, R. I. Estrogen use, hypertension and stroke in postmenopausal women. *Journal of Chronic Disease.* 1978; 31:389–98.

Pines, A., et al. The effects of hormone replacement therapy in normal postmenopausal women: Measurements of Doppler-derived parameters of aortic flow. *American Journal of Obstetrics and Gynecology.* March 1991; 164(3):806–12.

Powers, M. S., et al. Pharmacokinetics and pharmacodynamics of transdermal dosage forms of 17B estradiol: Comparison with conventional oral estrogens used for hormone replacement. *American Journal of Obstetrics and Gynecology.* 1985; 152:1099–106.

Psaty, B. M., et al. A review of the association of estrogens and progestins with cardiovascular disease in postmenopausal women. *Archives of Internal Medicine.* June 1993; 153(12):1421–7.

Quigley, M. E., et al. Estrogen therapy arrests bone loss in elderly women. *American Journal of Obstetrics and Gynecology.* 1987; 156:1516–23.

Raz, R., and W. E. Stamm. A controlled trial of intravaginal estriol in postmenopausal women with recurrent urinary tract infections. *New England Journal of Medicine.* September 1993; 329(11):753–6

Rigg, L. A., et al. Absorption of estrogen from vaginal creams. *New England Journal of Medicine.* 1976; 298:195–7.

Riss, B. J., et al. The effect of percutaneous estradiol and natural progesterone on postmenopausal bone loss. *American Journal of Obstetrics and Gynecology.* 1987; 156:61–5.

Ross, R. K., et al. Menopausal oestrogen therapy and protection from death from ischaemic heart disease. *Lancet.* 1981; 1:858–60.

Schiff, I., et al. Vaginal absorption of estrone and 17-B-estradiol. *Fertility and Sterility.* 1977; 28:1063–6.

Semmens, J. P. Postmenopausal vaginal physiology-effects of estrogen deprivation on sexual relations. *Clinical Practice in Sexuality.* 1986; 3(7):10–7.

Sherwin, B. B., and M. M. Gelfand. Differential symptom response to parenteral estrogen and/or androgen administration in the surgical menopause. *Obstetrics and Gynecology.* 1985; 151:153–60.

Sorrel, D. M. Sexuality and menopause. *Obstetrics and Gynecology.* 1990; 75:26S.

Spellacy, W. N. Menopause, estrogen treatment and carbohydrate metabolism. *Menopause. Yearbook Medical Publishers.* 1987; 256–8.

Speroff, L. Estrogen replacement today: A preventive health care issue. *Current Trends in Estrogen Replacement Therapy. HP Publishing.* 1986.

Stampfer, M. J., and G. A. Colditz. Estrogen replacement therapy and coronary heart disease: A quantitative assessment of the epidemiological evidence. *Preventive Medicine.* 1991; 20:47–63.

Steingold, K. A., et al. Treatment of hot flashes with transdermal estradiol administration. *Journal of Clinical Endocrinology & Metabolism.* 1985; 61:627.

Stevenson, J. C. Pathogenesis, prevention and treatment of osteoporosis. *Obstetrics and Gynecology.* 1990; 75:36S.

Storm, T., et al. Effects of intermittent cyclical etidronate therapy on bone mass and fracture rate in women with postmenopausal osteoporosis. *New England Journal of Medicine.* 1990; 322:1265–71.

Subbiah, M. T., et al. Antioxidant potential of specific estrogens on lipid peroxidation. *Journal of Clinical Endocrinology and Metabolism.* October 1993; 77(4):1095–7.

Utian, W. H. Biosynthesis and physiologic effects of estrogen and pathophysiologic effects of estrogen deficiency: A review. *American Journal of Obstetrics and Gynecology.* 1989; 161:1828–31.

Utian, W. H. Current perspectives in management of the menopausal and postmenopausal patient: Introduction. *Obstetrics and Gynecology*. 1990; 75:1S.

Vandenbroucke, J. P., et al. Noncontraceptive hormones and rheumatoid arthritis in perimenopausal and postmenopausal women. *Journal of the American Medical Association*. 1986; 255:1299–303.

Vandenbroucke, J. P. Oral contraceptives and rheumatoid arthritis in perimenopausal and postmenopausal women. *Journal of the American Medical Association*. 1986; 255:1299–303.

Watts, N. B., et al. Intermittent cyclical etidronate treatment of postmenopausal osteoporosis. *New England Journal of Medicine*. 1990; 323:73–9.

Weiss, N. S., et al. Endometrial cancer in relation to patterns of menopausal estrogen use. *Journal of the American Medical Association*. 1979; 242:261–4.

Wenger, N. K., et al. Cardiovascular Health and Disease in Women. New England Journal of Medicine. July 1993; 329(4):247–54.

Whitehead, M. I., et a. Transdermal administration of oestrogen/progestagen hormone replacement therapy. *Lancet*. 1990; 335:310–2.

Wilson, P. W. F., et al. Postmenopausal estrogen use, cigarette smoking, and cardiovascular morbidity in women over 50. *New England Journal of Medicine*. 1985; 313:1038–43.

Part II, Vitamins and Minerals, Books

Erasmus, U. *Fats and Oils*. Burnaby, BC, Canada: Alive Books, 1986.

Gittleman, A. L. *Supernutrition for Women*. New York: Bantam Books, 1991.

Hasslering, B., S. Greenwood, M.D., and M. Castleman. *The Medical Self-Care Book of Women's Health*. New York: Doubleday, 1987.

Hogladaroom, G., R. McCorkle, and N. Woods. *The Complete Book of Women's Health*. Englewood Cliff, NJ: Prentice Hall, 1982.

Kirschmann, J., and L. Dunne. *Nutrition Almanac*. New York: McGraw-Hill, 1984.

Kutsky, R. *Vitamins and Hormones*. New York: Van Nostrand Reinhold, 1973.

Lambert-Lagace, L. *The Nutrition Challenge for Women*. Palo Alto, CA. Bull Publishing Co., 1990.

Lark, S., M.D. *Fibroid Tumors and Endometriosis. A Self-Help Program*. Los Altos, CA: Westchester Publishing Co., 1993.

Lark, S., M.D. *Menopause Self-Help Book*. Berkeley, CA: Celestial Arts, 1992.

Padus, E. *The Woman's Encyclopedia of Health and Natural Healing*. Emmaus, PA: Rodale Press, 1981.

Reuben, C., and J. Priestly. *Essential Supplement for Women*. New York: Perigree Books, 1988.

Part II, Vitamins and Minerals, Articles

Albanese, A. A., et al. Effects of calcium supplements and estrogen replacement therapy on bone loss of postmenopausal women. *Nutrition Reports International* 1981; 24:404.

Anastasi, J., and M. Steiner. Effect of alpha-tocopherol on known platelet aggregation. *Division of Hematologic Research, The Memorial Hospital; Pawtucket and Brown University, RI* 1974.

Ant, M. Diabetic vulvovaginitis treated with vitamin E suppositories. *American Journal of Obstetrics and Gynecology* 1954; 67:407.

Band, P. R., et al. Treatment of benign breast disease with vitamin A. *Preventive Medicine* 1984; 13:549.

Biskind, M. S., and G. R. Biskind. Effect of vitamin B complex deficiency on inactivation of estrone in the liver. *Endocrinology* 1942; 31:109.

Biskind, M. S. Nutritional deficiency in the etiology of menorrhagia, cystic mastitis and premenstrual tension, treatment with vitamin B complex. *Journal of Clinical Endocrinology and Metabolism* 1943; 3:227.

Block, G. Vitamin C and cancer prevention. The epidemiologic evidence. *American Journal of Clinical Nutrition* 1991; 53:2701.

Boykin, L. S. Iron deficiency anemia in postmenopausal women. *Journal of the American Geriatrics Society* 1976; 24:558.

Brattstrom, L. E., et al. Folic acid responsive postmenopausal homocysteinemia. *Metabolism* 1985; 34:1073.

Breast Cancer Prevention Group. Breast cancer environmental factors. *The Lancet* 1992; 340:904.

Cheng, E. W., et al. Estrogenic activity of some naturally occurring isoflavones. *Annals of New York Academy of Sciences* 1955; 61(3):652.

Christy, C. J. Vitamin E in menopause. Preliminary report of experimental and clinical study. *American Journal of Obstetrics and Gynecology* 1945; 50:84.

Clemetson, C. A. B., et al. Capillary strength and the menstrual cycle. *New York Academy of Sciences* 1962; 93(7):277.

Cohen, J. D., and H. W. Rubin. Functional menorrhagia. Treatment with bioflavonoids and vitamin C. *Current Therapeutic Research* 1960; 2(11):539.

Cordova, C., et al. Influence of ascorbic acid on platelet aggregation in vitro and in vivo. *Atherosclerosis* 1981; 41:15.

Corson, S. L., and V. G. Upton. The perimenopause. Physiologic correlates and clinical management. *Journal of Reproductive Medicine* 1982; 27:1.

Dawson-Hughes, B., et al. A controlled trial of the effect of calcium supplementation on bone density in postmenopausal women. *New England Journal of Medicine* 1990; 323 (13):878.

Eskin, E. A., et al. Mammary gland dysplasia and iodine deficiency. *Journal of the American Medical Association* 1967; 200:115.

Finkler, R. S. The effect of vitamin E in the menopause. *Journal of Clinical Endocrinology* 1949; 9:89.

Frithiof, et al. The relationship between marginal bone loss and serum zinc levels. *ACTA Med Scand* 1980; 27:67.

Fuchs, N. K. Magnesium. The key to calcium absorption. *Let's Live* 1985.

Gallagher, J. C., and B. L. Riggs. Current concepts in nutrition. Nutrition and bone disease. *New England Journal of Medicine* 1978; 298:193.

Gallagher, J. C., et al. Intestinal calcium absorption and serum vitamin D metabolites in normal subjects and osteoporotic patients. *Journal of Clinical Investigation* 1979; 64:729.

Gerster, K. Potential role of beta carotene in the prevention of cardiovascular disease. *International Journal of Vitamin and Nutries Research* 1991; 61:277-91.

Goldin, B. R., et al. Effect of diet on excretion of estrogens in pre- and postmenopausal women. *Cancer Research* 1981; 41:3771.

Goldin, B. R., et al. Estrogen excretion patterns and plasma levels in vegetarian and omnivorous women. *New England Journal of Medicine* 1982; 307:1542.

Goodnight, S. H. The effects of Omega-3 fatty acids on thrombosis and atherogenesis. *Hematologic Pathology* 1989; 3(1):1.

Goodnight, S. H. Assessment of the therapeutic use of N-3 fatty acids in vascular disease and thrombosis *Chest*. 1991; 102(4):3745.

Gozan, H. A. The use of vitamin E in the treatment of menopause. *New York State Medical Journal* 1952; 15:1289.

Hain, A. M., and J. C. B. Sym. The control of menopausal flushes by vitamin E. *British Medicine Journal* 1943; 7:9.

Hasling, C., et al. Calcium metabolism in post menopausal osteoporotic women is determined by dietary calcium and coffee intake. *Journal of Nutrition* 1991; 112:1119-1126.

Haspels, et al. Estrogens and vitamin B6. *Frontiers of Hormone Research* 1975; 3:199.

Heaney, R. P., et al. Effect of calcium on skeletal development, bone loss and wrist fractures. *The American Journal of Medicine* 1991; 5B-23S—5B-28S.

Hennekens, C. A., et al. Beta carotene and cardiovascular disease. Beyond deficiency. New views on the functions and health effects of vitamins. *New York Academy of Sciences*. 1992; 22.

Henson, D. L., et al. Ascorbic acid. Biological functions and relation to cancer. *Journal of The National Cancer Institute* 1991; 83(8):547-50.

Hollander, D., and A. Tarmawski. Dietary essential fatty acids and the decline in peptic ulcer disease. *Gut* 1986; 22(3):239.

Horrobin, D. F. Essential fatty acid and prostaglandin metabolism in Sjogren's Syndrome. Systemic sclerosis and rheumatoid arthritis. *Scandinavian Journal of Rheumatology Supplement* 1980; 61:242.

Horrobin, D. F. Essential fatty acids and the complications of diabetes mellitus. *Wien Klin Wochenschr* 1989; 101(8):289.

Horrobin, D. F. Essential fatty acids in clinical dermatology. *Journal of the American Academy of Dermatology* 1987 20(6):1045.

Horrobin, D. F. The regulation of prostaglandin biosynthesis by the manipulation of essential fatty acid metabolism. *Revue of Pure and Applied Pharmacologic Science* 1980; 4(4):339.

Horsman, A., et al. Prospective trial of oestrogen and calcium in postmenopausal women. *British Medial Journal* 1977; 2:789.

Howe, G. R., et al. Dietary factors and the risk of breast cancer. Combined analysis of 12 case-controlled studies. *Journal of The National Cancer Institute* 1990; 82:561-9.

Hunter, D. T. Antioxidant micronutrients and breast cancer. *Journal of the American College of Nutrition* 1992; 11(5):633.

Jowsey, J. Osteoporosis. Its nature and the role of diet. *Postgraduate Medicine* 1976; 60(2):75.

Kavinovsky, N. R. Vitamin E and the control of climacteric symptoms. *Annals of Western Medicine and Surgery* 1950; 4(1):27.

Kellis, T., and L. E. Vickery. Inhibition of human estrogen synthetase (aromatase) by flavones. *Science* 1984; 225:1032-4.

Kruse, C. A. Treatment of fatigue with aspartic acid salts. *Northwest Medicine* 1961; 6:597.

Lee, C. J., et al. Effects of supplementation of the diets with calcium and calcium rich food on bone density of elderly females with osteoporosis. *American Journal of Clinical Nutrition* 1981; 34:819.

Licato, A. Effect of supplemental calcium on serum and urinary calcium in osteoporotic patients. *Journal of the American College of Nutrition* 1992; 11(2):164-7.

Lindquist, O. Influence of the menopause on ischemic heart disease and its risk factors and on bone mineral content. *ACTA Obstetrica et Gynecologica Scandinavica* 1982; 110:7.

Lithgow, P. M., and W. M. Politzer. Vitamin A in the treatment of menorrhagia. *South African Medical Journal* 1977; 51:191.

London, R. S., et al. Endocrine parameters in alpha-tocopheryl therapy of patients with mammary dysplasia. *Cancer Research* 1981; 41:3811.

London, R. S., et al. Mammary dysplasia. Clinical response and urinary excretion of 11-deoxy-17-ketosteroids and pregnanediol following alpha-tocopherol therapy. *Breast* 1976; 4:19.

Lutz, J. Calcium balance and acid base status of women as affected by increased protein intake and by sodium bicarbonate ingestion. *American Journal of Clinical Nutrition* 1984; 39:20.

Machtey, I., and L. Ouaknine. Tocopherol in osteoarthritis. A controlled pilot study. *Journal of the American Geriatrics Society* 1978; 26:328.

Manku, M. S., et al. Prolactin and zinc effects on rat vascular ractivity. Possible relationship to dihomogammalinolenic acid and to prostaglandin synthesis. *Endocrinology* 1979; 104:774.

Mansel, R. E., et al. The use of evening primrose oil in mastalgia. *Clinical Uses of Essential Fatty Acids* 1983.

Manson, T., et al. A prospective study of vitamin C and the incidence of coronary heart disease in women. *Circulation* 1992; 85:865.

Marcus, R. The relationship of dietary calcium to maintenance of skeletal integrity of man. An interface of endocrinology and nutrition. *Metabolism* 1982; 31:93.

McKeown, L. A. Diet high in fruits and vegetables linked to lower breast cancer risk. *Medical Tribune* 1992; 9:14.

McLaren, H. C. Vitamin E in the menopause. *British Medical Journal* 1949; 12:1378.

Nicholson, J. P., and C. M. Resnick. Outpatient therapy of essential hypertension with dietary calcium supplementation. *Journal of the American College of Cardiology* 1984; 2:616.

Osilesi, O., et al. Blood pressure and plasma lipids during ascorbic acid supplementation to borderline hypertensive and normotensive adults. *Nutrition Research* 1991; 11:405-12.

Pauling, L. Prevention and treatment of heart disease. New research focus at the Linus Pauling Institute. *Linus Pauling Institute of Science and Medicine Newsletter* 1992; 1.

Pauling, L. How vitamin C can prevent heart attack and stroke. *Linus Pauling Institute for Science and Medicine Newsletter* 1992; 3.

Pauling, L. Vitamin C and heart disease. A chronology. *Linus Pauling Institute for Science and Medicine Newsletter* 1992; 2.

Pope, G. S., et al. Isolation of oestrogenic isoflavone (biochanin A) from red clover. *Chemistry and Industry* 1953; 10:1042.

Potischman, N. Association between breast cancer, plasma triglycerides and cholesterol. *Nutrition and Cancer* 1991; 15:205-15.

Preuter, G. W. A treatment for excessive uterine bleeding. *Applied Therapeutics* 1961; 5:351.

Renaud, S., and L. McGregor. Essential fatty acids and the platelet membrane in relation to aggregation. *Annals de la Nutrition de l'Alimentation* 1980; 34(2):265.

Riggs, L., et al. Treatment of primary osteoporosis with fluoride and calcium. Clinical tolerance and fracture occurrence. *Journal of the American Medical Association* 1987; 243:446.

Rude, R. K., et al. Low serum concentrations of 1.25-dihydroxyvitamin D in human magnesium deficiency. *Journal of Clinical Endocrinology and Metabolism* 1985; 61:933.

Schrauzer, G. N., et al. Selenium in the blood of Japanese and American women with and without breast cancer and fibrocystic disease. *Japanese Journal of Cancer Research* 1985; 76:374.

Seelig, M. S. The requirements of magnesium by the normal adult. *American Journal of Clinical Nutrition* 1964; 14:342.

Shute, E. V., et al. The influence of vitamin E on vascular disease. *Surgery, Gynecology and Obstetrics* 1948; 86:1.

Simard, A. Nutrition and lifestyle factors in fibrocystic disease and cancer of the breast. *Cancer Prevention and Nutrition* 1990; 567-72.

Simin, T. Vitamin C and cardiovascular disease. A review. *The American College* of Nutrition 1992; 11(2):107-25.

Singer, E. Effects of vitamin E deficiency on the thyroid gland of the rat. *Journal of Physiology* 1936; 87:287.

Skrabel, F., et al. Low sodium/high potassium diet for prevention of hypertension. Probable mechanisms of action. *Lancet* 1981; 10:895.

Smith, C. J. Nonhormonal control of vaso-motor flushing in menopausal patients. *Chicago Medicine* 1964; 67:193.

Solomon, D., et al. Relationship between vitamin E and urinary excretion of ketosteroid fractions in cystic mastitis. *Annals of New York Academy of Sciences* 1972; 2(3):103.

Stone, K. J., et al. The metabolism of dihomogammalineolenic acid in man. *Lipids* 1979; 14:174.

Takeda, S. Liquid peroxidation in human breast cancer cells in response to gamma-linolenic acid and iron. *Anticancer Research* 1992.12:329-34.

Taylor, F. A. Habitual abortion. Therapeutic evaluation of citrus bioflavonoids. *Western Journal of Surgery, Obstetrics and Gynecology* 1956; 5:286.

Taymor, M. L., et al. The etiological role of chronic iron deficiency in production of menorrhagia. *Journal of the American Medical Association* 1964; 187:323.

Taymor, M. L., et al. Menorrhagia due to chronic iron deficiency. *Obstetrics and Gynecology* 1960; 16:571.

Van Beresteijn, E. Habitual dietary calcium intake and cortical bone loss in perimenopausal women. A longitudinal study. *Calcified Tissue International* 1990; 47:338-44.

Vles, R. O. Essential fatty acids in cardiovascular physiopathology. *Annales de la Nutrition et de l'Alimentation* 1980; 34(2):255.

Watson, E. M. Clinical experiences with wheat germ oil (vitamin E). *Canadian Medical Association Journal* 1936; 2:134.

Weaver, C. M. Calcium bioavailability and its relationship to osteoporosis. *Proceedings for the Society of Experimental Biology and Medicine* 1992; 200:157-60.

Wertz, P. W., et al. Essential fatty acids and epidermal integrity. *Archives of Dermatology* 1987; 123(10):1381.

Whitacre, F. E., and B. Barrera. War amenorrhea. *Journal of the American Medical Association* 1944; 124:399.

Wilcox, G., et al. Estrogen effects of plant foods in postmenopausal women. *British Medical Journal* 1990; 301:905-6.

Wiley-Rosett, J. A., et al. Influence of vitamin A on cervical dysplasia and carcinoma in situ. *Nutrition and Cancer* 1984; 6(1):49.

Zardize, D. G. Fatty acid composition of phospholipids in erythrocyte membranes and risk of breast cancer. *International Journal of Cancer* 1990; 45:807-10.

Part II, Herbs, Books

Castleman, M. *The Healing Herbs*. Emmaus, PA: Rodale Press, 1991.

Colbin, A. *Food and Healing*. New York: Ballantine Books, 1986.

Hasselbring, B., et al. *The Medical Self-Care Book of Women's Health*. New York: Doubleday, 1987.

Hylton, W. *The Rodale Herb Booke*. Emmaus, PA: Rodale Press, 1974.

Lark, S. *Menopause Self-Help Book*. Berkeley, CA: Celestial Arts, 1992.

Lust, J. *The Herb Book*. New York: Bantam, 1974.

Mowrey, D. *The Scientific Validation of Herbal Medicine*. New Canaan, CT: Keats Publishing, 1986.

Murray, M. *The 21st Century Herbal, Volume I*. Bellevue, WA: Vita-Line, 1985.

Murray, M. *The 21st Century Herbal, Volume II*. Bellevue, WA: Vita-Line, 1985.

Padus, E. *The Woman's Encyclopedia of Health and Natural Healing*. Emmaus, PA: Prevention Books, 1981.

Rector-Page, L. *How to be Your Own Herbal Pharmacist*. Linda Rector-Page, Pub., 1991.

Part II, Herbs, Articles

Ammon, H. P. T., and A. B. Muller. Forskolin: From ayurvedic remedy to a modern agent. *Planta Medica* 1985; 51:473-7.

Baranov, A. I. Medicinal uses of ginseng and related plants in the Soviet Union: Recent trends in the Soviet literature. *Journal of Ethnopharmacology* 1982; 6:339-53.

Butler, C. L., and C. H. Costello. Pharmacologic studies. I. Aletris farinosa. *Journal of the American Pharmaceutical Society* 1944. 33:177-83.

Costello, C. H., and E. V. Lynn. Estrogenic substances from plants. I. Glycyrrhiza. *Journal of the American Pharmaceutical Society* 1950. 39:177-80.

Chang, J., et al. Effect of forskolin on prostanglanding synthesis by mouse resident peritoneal macrophages. *European Journal of Pharmacology* 1984. 103:303-12

Chen, E. W., et al. Estrogenic activity of some naturally occurring isoflavones. *Annals of the New York Academy of Sciences* 1955. 61(3):652

Cohen, J. D., and H. W. Rubin. Functional menorrhagia: Treatment with bioflavonoids and vitamin C. *Current Therapeutic Research* 1960. 2(11):539.

Dansi, A., et al. The estrogenic activity of polymerized anol. *Biochimica e Terapia Sperimentale* 1937. 24:282-4.

Dodds, E. C., and W. Lawson. Estrogenic activity of p-hydroxypropenyl-benzene (anol). *Nature* 1937. 139:1039.

Dodds, E. C., and W. Lawson. A simple oestrogenic agent with an activity of the same order as that of oestrone. *Nature* 1937. 139:627.

Elghamry, M. I., and I. M. Shihata. Biological activity of phytoestrogens. *Planta Medica* 1965. 13:352-7.

Faber, K. The dandelion-Taraxacum officinale weber. *Pharmazie* 1958. 13:423-35.

Gibson, M. R. Glycyrrhiza in old and new perspectives. *Lloydia* 1978. 41:348-54.

Gomez, E. T., and C. W. Turner. Effect of anol and dihydrotheelin on mammogenic activity of the pituitary gland of rabbits. *Proceedings of the Society for Experimental Biology and Medicine* 1938. 39:140-42.

Hahn, F. E., and J. Ciak. Berberine. *Antibiotics* 1976. 3:577-88.

Harada, M., et al. Effect of Japanese angelica root and peony root on uterine contraction in the rabbit in situ. *Journal of Pharmacologic Dynamics* 1984. 7:304-11.

Havsteen, B. Flavonoids, a class of natural products of high pharmacological potency. *Biochemical Pharmacology* 1983. 32:1141-8.

Kerouac, R., et al. Forskolin inhibits histamine release by neurotension in the rat perfused hind limb. *Research Communications Chemical Pathology Pharmacology* 1984. 45:310-2.

Kuhnau, J. The flavonoids: A class of semi-essential food components: Their role in human nutrition. *World Review of Nutrition and Diet* 1976. 24:117-91.

Leathwood, P. D., and F. Chauffard. Aqueous extract of valerian reduces latency to fall asleep in man. *Planta Medica* 1985. 54:144-8.

Leathwood, P. D., et al. Aqueous extract of valerian root (Valeriani Officinalis L.) improves sleep quality in man. *Pharmacol. Biochem Behavior* 1982. 17:65-71.

Middleton, E. The flavonoids. *Trends in Pharmaceutical Science* 1984. 5:335-8.

Pearse, H. A., and J. D. Trisler. A rational approach to the treatment of habitual abortion and menometorrhagia. *Clinical Medicine* 1957. 9:1081.

Pope, G. S., et al. Isolation of an oestrogenic isoflavone (Biochanin A) from red clover. *Chemistry and Industry* 1953. 10:1042.

Potter, D. E., et al. Forskolin suppresses sympathetic neuron function and causes ocular hypotension. *Current Eye Research* 1985. 4:87-96.

Preuter, G. W. A treatment for excessive uterine bleeding. *Applied Therapeutics* 1961. 5:351.

Racz-Kotilla, E., et al. The action of taraxacum offinale extracts on the body weight and diuresis of laboratory animals. *Planta Medica* 1974. 26:212-7.

Sabir, M., and N. Bhide. Study of some pharmacologic actions of berberine. *Indian Journal of Physical Pharmacology* 1971. 15:111-32.

Schumann, E. Newer concepts of blood coagulation and control of hemorrhage. *American Journal of Obstetrics and Gynecology* 1939. 38:1002-7.

Suekawa, M., et al. Pharmacological studies on ginger. I. pharmacological actions of pungent constituents, (6) gingerol and (6) shogaol. *Journal of Pharmacologic Dynamics* 1984. 7:836-48.

Tanaka, S., et al. Antinociceptive substances from the roots of angelica acutiloga. *Arzneim-Forsch* 1977. 27:2039-45.

Taylor, F. A. Habitual abortion: Therapeutic evaluation of citrus bioflavonoids. *Western Journal of Surgery, Obstetrics and Gynecology* 1956. 5:280.

Part II, Stress Reduction

Benson, R., and M. Klipper. *Relaxation Response*. New York: Avon, 1976.

Bourne, E. J. *The Anxiety and Phobia Workbook*. Oakland, CA: New Harbinger Publications, 1990

Brennan, B. A. *Hands of Light*. New York: Bantam, 1987.

Davis, M. M., M. Eshelman, and E. Eshelman. *The Relaxation and Stress-reduction Workbook*. Oakland, CA: New Harbinger Publications, 1982.

Gawain, S. *Creative Visualization*. San Rafael, CA: New World Publishing, 1978.

Gawain, S. *Living in the Light*. Mill Valley, CA: Whatever Publishing, 1986.

Kripalu Center for Holistic Health. *The Self-Health Guide*. Lenox, MA: Kripalu Publications, 1980.

Loehr, J., and J. Migdow. *Take a Deep Breath*. New York: Villard Books, 1986.

Miller, E. *Self-Imagery*. Berkeley, CA: Celestial Arts, 1986.

Ornstein, R., and D. Sobel. *Healthy Pleasures*. Reading, MA: Addison-Wesley, 1989.

Padis, E. *Your Emotions and Your Health*. Emmaus, PA: Rodale Press, 1986.

Part II,
Exercise and Menopause Relief, Books

Bailey, C. *Fit or Fat?* Boston: Houghton Miffen, 1977.

Bauer, C. *Acupressure for Women.* Freedom, CA: The Crossing Press, 1987.

Bell, L., and E. Seyfer. *Gentle Yoga.* Berkeley, CA: Celestial Arts, 1987.

Caillet, R., M.D., and C. Gross. *The Rejuvenation Strategy.* New York: Pocket Books, 1987.

Chang, S. *The Complete Book of Acupuncture.* Berkeley, CA: Celestial Arts, 1976.

Couch, J., and N. Weaver. *Runner's World Yoga Book.* New York: Runner's World Books, 1979.

Folan, L. *Lilias, Yoga, and Your Life.* New York: McMillan Publishing Co., 1981.

Gach, M. R., and C. Marco. *Acu-Yoga.* Tokyo: Japan Publications, 1981

Hanna, T. *Somatics.* Reading, MA: Addison-Wesley Publishing Co., Inc., 1988.

Houston, F. M. *The Healing Benefits of Acupressure.* New Canaan, CT: Keats Publishing, 1974.

Huang, C. A. *Tai Ji.* Berkeley, CA: Celestial Arts, 1989.

Iyengar, B. K. S. *Light on Yoga.* New York: Schocken Books, 1966.

Jerome, J. *Staying Supple.* New York: Bantam Books, 1987.

Kenyon, J. *Acupressure Techniques.* Rochester, VT. Healing Arts Press, 1980.

Kripalu Center for Holistic Health. *The Self-Help Guide.* Lenox, MA: Kripalu Publications, 1980.

McLish, R., and J. Vedral, PhD. *Perfect Parts.* New York: Warner Books, 1987.

Mittleman, R. *Yoga 28 Day Exercise Plan.* New York: Workman Publishing Co., 1969.

Moore, M., and M. Douglas. *Yoga.* Arcane, ME: Arcane Publications, 1967.

Nickel, D. J. *Acupressure for Athletes.* New York: Henry Holt, 1984

Pendleton, B., and B. Mehling. *Relax With Self-Therap/Ease.* Englewood Cliffs, NJ: Prentice-Hall, 1984.

Pinkney, C. *Callanetics: 10 Years Younger in 10 Hours.* New York: Avon, 1984.

Singh, R. *Kundalini Yoga.* New York: White Lion Press, 1988.

Solveborn, S. A., M.D. *The Book About Stretching.* New York: Japan Publications, 1985.

Stearn, J. *Yoga, Youth and Reincarnation.* New York: Bantam, 1965.

Teeguarden, I. *Acupressure Way of Health. Jin Shin Do.* Tokyo: Japan Publications, 1978.

The Academy of Traditional Chinese Medicine. *An Outline of Chinese Acupuncture.* New York: Pergamon Press, 1975.

Tobias, M., and M. Stewart. *Stretch and Relax.* Tucson, AZ: The Body Press, 1985.

Index

nutrition and, 116, 124, 128, 130, 131, 132, 139, 173–75, 189
See also specific types of cancer
Carbohydrate metabolism, 117, 182–83
Cardiovascular disease, 111–20
  acupressure for, 283–84, 285
  caffeine and, 134
  cause of heart attacks, 111
  described, 111, 119
  estrogen and, 15, 116
  exercise and, 241–43, 266
  herbs for, 206–08, 210
  hormone replacement therapy and, 31, 36, 45, 52, 58, 117–20
  hypertension and, 114
  incidence of, 111, 119, 129
  nutrition and, 116, 129, 130, 131, 132, 134, 139, 169, 186–88
  postmenopausal, 19, 116
  potassium caution, 181
  risk factors for, 112–16, 119, 120
Carrots, 130, 131, 153, 156, 171, 173
Casseroles, 164, 166, 167, 207
CAT (computerized axial tomography) scans, 101
Catecholamines, 88–89
Cereals, 136, 150–52
Cervical cancer, 131, 173–74
Cervical sensitivity, 77–78, 81
Cheese, 147, 161, 164. *See also* Dairy products
Chest expander, 263–65
Chocolate, 84, 133–35, 162, 168. *See also* Caffeine
Cholesterol, 15, 52, 113–14
  herbs for, 207
  hormone replacement therapy and, 34–35, 45, 58
  nutrition and, 126, 127, 131, 134, 139
  See also Lipids
Chromium, 182–83, 191
Cigarettes. *See* Smoking
Clitoral enlargement, androgens and, 31
Clitoral sensitivity, 77–78, 81
Clonidine, 73

Clotting problems. *See* Blood clotting problems
Coffee. *See* Caffeine
Cola drinks, 133–35, 136, 137. *See also* Caffeine
Colon cancer, 128, 139, 186
Condoms, 85
Constipation, 127, 132–33
Copper, 126, 191
Corn, 126–28
Corpus luteum, 12, 15, 17
Cortisone, osteoporosis and, 100
Counseling services, 93
Cramps, 66, 202, 214–17, 257–60
Cravings, food, 62, 128, 137
Creams
  skin, 35, 37, 65–66
  vaginal, 29–31, 51–52, 53, 80, 81–82, 86, 104
  See also Gels
Crying, 179, 211
CVAs (cerebral vascular accidents). *See* Cardiovascular disease
Cystocele, 80

Dairy products
  risks of, 130, 139–40, 141
  substitutes, 84, 85–86, 133, 141, 164–65, 168
Dalmane, 91
D&C (dilation and curettage), 64
Dementia, 44
Densitometers, 101
Depo-Provera, 72
Depression
  acupressure for, 278–79, 285
  alcohol and, 135
  exercise and, 238–39, 266
  herbs for, 205–06, 210
  hormone replacement therapy and, 2, 33, 34, 37, 43–44, 57, 90
  hormones and, 16, 88
  hysterectomies and, 42
  menopause and, 62, 87, 88, 211
  mood-altering drugs for, 91–93
  neurotransmitters and, 92
  nutrition and, 128, 135, 179, 180, 181
  See also Relaxation techniques

DES (diethylstilbestrol), 26
Desserts, 133, 136, 137, 145, 166. *See also* Chocolate; Sugar
Diabetes, 52, 53–54, 114, 136–37, 242
nutrition and, 125–26, 128, 130, 136–37, 182–83
supplements caution, 176, 179–80
Diet. *See* Nutrition
Dieting, 109, 242–43
Digestive tract, 27, 190, 205, 209, 249, 257–59
Dilation and curettage (D&C), 64
Dizziness, 70, 171
Douching, 85
Dowager's hump, 95, 98–99
Drowsiness, progesterone replacement therapy and, 35
Drugs
addiction to, 239
for hot flashes, 72–73
mood-altering, 91–93
for osteoporosis, 105, 108
See also Androgens; Estrogen replacement therapy; Progesterone replacement therapy; *specific drugs*
Dual x-ray absorptiometry, 24

Eating disorders, 100, 183
Edema, salt and, 138
Eggs (human). *See* Follicles; Ovaries
Eicosapentaenoic acid (EPA), 130
Elavil, 92
Electrolysis, 109
Emotions
estrogen replacement therapy and, 22, 36, 43–44, 47, 90–91
exercise and, 237–39
hot flashes and, 71
menopause and, 44, 211–12
nutrition and, 47, 57, 134, 135, 137, 145, 172, 177–83
progesterone replacement therapy and, 33, 34, 37, 57
See also Anger; Anxiety; Depression; Irritability; Mood swings; Nervous tension; Relaxation techniques

Endometriosis, 54, 171
Endometrium
biopsies of, 64, 65
cancer of. *See* Uterine cancer
hyperplasia of, 24, 48, 64–65, 81–82
menstrual cycle and, 12–13
ERT. *See* Estrogen replacement therapy
Essential fatty acids. *See* Fatty acids
Estrace, 26
Estraderm, 28
Estradiol, 13, 14, 25, 26, 127
Estriol, 13–14, 25, 26, 86, 127
Estrogel, 32
Estrogen. *See individual topics*
Estrogen replacement therapy (ERT), 21–74. *See individual topics*
Estrone, 13, 14, 25, 26, 68, 127
Evening primrose oil, 176–77
Exercise, 233–48

Facial drooping, 102
Facial hair, 17, 31, 82, 103, 107
Faintness, 70, 171
Fallopian tubes, 12, 15, 16
Family history, 98–99, 112
Family relationships. *See* Relationships
Fast food, 138, 144–45, 147
Fat (body), 15, 19, 46, 49, 99, 112. *See also* Weight
Fat (dietary), 14, 50–51, 52, 116, 127, 129, 139–41. *See also* Fatty acids
Fatigue
alcohol and, 135
hormone replacement therapy and, 33, 34, 37, 43–44, 90
hysterectomies and, 42
menopause and, 62, 87, 88, 211
mood-altering drugs for, 92
nutrition and, 128, 132, 133, 135, 145, 164
vitamins and minerals, 171, 173, 177, 178–79, 180–82
postmenopausal, 19
progesterone and, 16, 88
Fatty acids, 128–30, 176–77, 188

Spinal exercises, 255–56, 257–59, 260–61
Spinal fractures, 95, 105, 108
Spotting, 38, 46, 63
STDs (sexually transmitted diseases), 85
Stilbestrol, 203
Stopping hormone use, 39, 46
Stress
    exercise and, 234, 235, 241–42, 247, 259–60
    herbs for, 205–06, 210
    negative effects of, 71, 88–89, 115
    nutrition and, 177–83
    See also Relaxation techniques
Stress incontinence, 80, 81, 107
Strokes. *See* Cardiovascular disease
Subcutaneous estrogen pellets, 32
Substituting healthy ingredients, 161–68
Sugar, 136–37
    negative effects of, 14, 84, 128, 136–37, 163
    substitutes, 133, 137, 163, 168
Sun exposure, skin and, 103, 109
Supplements, 169–99, 201–10. *See also* Fatty acids; Herbs; Minerals; Vitamins
Support groups, 93
Suppositories, progesterone, 35
Sweat glands, menopause and, 103. *See also* Night sweats
Sweeteners, 136, 141, 163, 168. *See also* Sugar
Synthetic estrogen, 26
Synthetic progesterone, 33–34, 37, 38, 56–57, 65, 72

Tablets, estrogen, 25–27
Tea
    black. *See* Caffeine
    herbal, 135, 162
Teeth, osteoporosis and, 95, 101–02
Temperature, 16, 103
Tension. *See* Muscle tension; Nervous tension
Testosterone, 9, 16–17, 47, 78, 82, 90–91, 97. *See also* Androgens

Thrombophlebitis. *See* Blood clotting problems
Thymus gland, 227
Thyroid gland, 11, 100, 131–32, 227, 243, 251
Thyroid hormones, 47, 96, 105, 234
Tingling, 70, 92
Tiredness. *See* Fatigue
Tofranil, 92
Trace minerals, 131–32, 167, 182, 185, 191, 206–07
Tranquilizers, 26, 73, 91, 92
Transdermal estrogen, 28–29, 36, 37, 51, 52, 53, 72, 80, 82, 104
Tricyclics, 92
Triglycerides, 113, 117, 134, 188
Tryptophan, 178, 204

Ultrasound, 64–65
Urethral prolapse, 107
Urinary incontinence, 80, 81, 107
Urinary tract, 15, 79, 85–86. *See also* Vaginal and bladder aging
Urinary tract infections, 29–30, 43, 78–79, 85–86, 204, 235
Uterine cancer, 13, 49, 64
    estrogen replacement therapy and, 2, 23, 27, 31, 34, 38, 48–49, 55
    progesterone replacement therapy and, 23, 27, 31, 33, 34, 35, 37, 38, 48–49, 55
Uterine polyps, 64
Uterine prolapse, 80, 107
Uterus
    growth and development of, 15
    menstrual cycle and, 12–13
    See also Fibroid tumors

Vagina, growth and development of, 15
Vaginal and bladder aging, 75–85, 86
    acupressure for, 281–82, 285
    alcohol and, 135
    described, 75–76
    exercise and, 235–37, 256–57, 266
    herbs for, 203–04, 208, 209

Middlebury College
Library

Middlebury Community
316 Library